CORONARY CARE UNIT NURSING:

A Workbook in Clinical Aspects

CORONARY CARE UNIT NURSING:

A Workbook in Clinical Aspects

Harold A. Braun, M.D.
Gerald A. Diettert, M.D.

 Reston Publishing Company, Inc.
A Prentice-Hall Company
Reston, Virginia

Library of Congress Cataloging in Publication Data

Braun, Harold A
  Coronary care unit nursing, a workbook in clinical
aspects.

  Includes bibliographical references and index.
  1. Coronary heart disease—Nursing.   2. Coronary
care units.   I. Diettert, Gerald A., joint author.
II. Title. [DNLM: 1. Coronary care units.   2. Coronary Disease—Nursing. WY152.5 B825]
RC685. C6B72   610.73'691   80-11052
ISBN 0-8359-1051-2

© 1980 by
Reston Publishing Company, Inc.
Reston, Virginia 22090
A Prentice-Hall Company

10 9 8 7 6 5 4 3 2 1

Printed in the United States of America

Contents

Acknowledgements

Early drafts of some of this material were prepared while planning the coronary care facilities of St. Patrick Hospital, Missoula, Montana. Additional material grew out of the Training Program for Intensive Coronary Care, conducted by the Mountain States Regional Medical Program, an activity of the Western Interstate Commission for Higher Education (Grant No. 1 GO3 RM-00032-01).

We appreciate the help and stimulation of many people, especially the nurses of the Special Care Unit of St. Patrick Hospital and Vera Wills, R.N. and Lillian La Croix, R.N.; the Cardiology Department of the Western Montana Clinic, and particularly Drs. Walter J. Lewis, W. Stan Wilson, and George H. Reed for their suggestions and criticisms.

HB and GD

Introduction

The nurse is the key person in the team providing intensive coronary care.

Training for coronary care nursing is difficult because some of the subject matter is difficult, because much of the subject matter is new to trainee and instructor alike, and because teaching materials are scarce. In addition, coronary care training is particularly difficult to provide precisely where it is needed most—in the hospital without a complex program of continuing education.

This text represents part of a continuing effort to develop materials useful for coronary care training. Because of our special interest in hospitals newly active in training, emphasis is given to practical details infrequently discussed. Other subjects, such as details of cardiopulmonary resuscitation, are presented with such frequency and excellence elsewhere that detail here is unnecessary.

STUDY SUGGESTIONS

Coronary Care Unit Nursing omits items best dealt with in the classroom or amply presented elsewhere, as indicated in the lists of *Suggested Reading*.

A question section closes most chapters. Although some questions may be difficult to answer solely on the basis of material presented in this book, they will suggest what the competent student will want to have assimilated on that topic, either from this text, lecture material, or collateral reading. The utility of this book will be greatest if used in conjunction with a formal curriculum of lectures and demonstrations. The instructor should indicate which section will be covered in a given lecture. *Before* the lecture, study this portion. *After* the lecture, complete the question section. If a question is difficult, the subject has not been made clear either within the text or in the lecture. This should be the first item for discussion at the next class session.

Coronary heart disease

Atherosclerosis is the principal form of *arteriosclerosis* (artery hardening), a disease involving the arteries. Atherosclerosis is characterized by the accumulation of fatty materials (lipids) beneath the inner lining *(intima)* of the walls of medium and large arteries. The major lipid deposition is *cholesterol*. The process, associated with scarring, deposition of calcium, and a reduction in the lumen of the artery is spotty in the form of *plaques*.

Atherosclerotic disease involves most often the coronary arteries, the aorta, and the cerebral, renal and peripheral arteries, and produces its clinical picture by a reduction in blood flow to the tissue *(ischemia)*. Ischemia may develop gradually as the plaque encroaches on the lumen of the artery. A blood clot *(thrombus)* may form in the lumen of an artery narrowed by a plaque, which may lead to interruption of blood flow to the tissues *(infarction)* and tissue death *(necrosis)*. The terms *coronary thrombosis* or *occlusion* are sometimes used to describe this event in a coronary artery.

Coronary heart disease has become the greatest sustained epidemic that man has experienced. It has been estimated that 3.1 million adults in the United States have definite coronary heart disease and another 2.4 million are suspect, together representing 5% of the adult population. Annually over one million heart attacks occur in the United States, with over 600,000 deaths.

About half die in the first few hours, often before medical care has been obtained. About 25% of those with first attacks die within 3 hours, and another 10% in the first weeks. Of those who survive, the death rate in the next five years is five times that of those without coronary heart disease, and death is usually due to another coronary episode. About 165,000 coronary deaths are in persons under age 65, predominantly men (3 to 1). The costs of this epidemic, estimated at $50 billion, are a major factor in the high cost of medical care. Annual mortality rates have shown some decrease in recent years.

RISK FACTORS

The cause of coronary atherosclerosis is unknown, but certain factors commonly are associated with the disease. Factors which increase the risk of coronary atherosclerosis include:

    A.   Hypertension
    B.   High serum cholesterol
    C.   Cigarette smoking
    D.   Diabetes
    E.   Heredity
    F.   Obesity
    G.   Sedentary living
    H.   Certain personality traits

Several studies indicate that the major risk factors in the development of premature coronary heart disease are high serum cholesterol, hypertension, and cigarette smoking. Middle-aged American males with none of these risk factors have much lower coronary morbidity and mortality rates than men with two or three of these factors. It is hoped that early identification of persons with risk factors and modification of them will lead to progress in preventing atherosclerotic diseases.

"PREHOSPITAL CARE"

Major emphasis has been directed toward care of the patient who develops clinical coronary heart disease in the form of myocardial infarction and sudden death. Since 50 to 65% of all heart-attack victims die within the first few hours, some communities have developed "early coronary care systems." Pioneered in Belfast, North Ireland, and further pursued by cities such as Seattle, Miami, New York City, Newark, and Columbus, Ohio, these systems employ mobile coronary care units containing emergency medication and battery-powered monitors and defibrillators. They are staffed by trained personnel such as firemen, ambulance drivers or hospital house staff. Over a decade's experience has demonstrated that many lives can be saved by these units. Hundreds of units are now in operation and many more are in the planning stages.

CORONARY CARE

The coronary care unit originally was developed to permit prompt treatment of cardiac arrest. It was soon recognized that monitoring allowed prompt recognition and treatment of minor arrhythmias, thus preventing catastrophic arrhythmias. Presently, the goal of intensive coronary care is the prevention of serious arrhythmias by early recognition and treatment of the minor arrhythmias which often precede them. In addition, efforts in the coronary care unit are now aimed toward preserving viable myocardium. Myocardial infarction results in necrosis (death) of some myocardial cells while cells in the surrounding area are ischemic but remain alive, though often with poor function. Under adverse conditions, some of these cells may also become necrotic. Therapy directed toward salvaging these ischemic cells by reducing myocardial work and oxygen consumption is now an important function of the coronary care unit. Chapter 7 discusses this in detail.

Currently, the coronary care unit is often used for other purposes such as: (1) monitoring of patients with arrhythmia problems without myocardial infarction; (2) monitoring of patients before and after pacemaker insertion; and (3) close observation of patients for whom it is important to monitor parameters such as cardiac rhythm, systemic blood pressure, pulmonary artery and pulmonary capillary wedge pressures, and central venous pressure.

Difficult decisions may develop when there is a bed shortage. Patients with severe myocardial damage resulting in congestive heart failure or shock require extensive care, though their prognosis is poor and their mortality rate has been little changed by current coronary intensive care. New techniques using drugs salvage only a small percentage of patients. Patients requiring intra-aortic balloon pumping rarely survive unless a definitive surgical procedure such as coronary artery-vein bypass graft, mitral valve replacement, or aneurysmectomy can be performed. (See Chapter 8).

CLINICAL CORONARY HEART DISEASE

The heart receives its blood supply from two coronary arteries which surround it like a "corona" or crown. About 5% of the heart's output is used to nourish the heart by these arteries. The distribution of the coronary arteries is variable. In about half of the population, the right coronary artery predominates, supplying the right ventricle and posterior left ventricle. The left coronary artery with its two major branches, the anterior descending and circumflex arteries, supplies the anterior and lateral left ventricle. In a third of the population, the arteries are "balanced," the right coronary artery supplying the right ventricle and part of the posterior left ventricle, and the left coronary artery supplying the remainder. Less often, the left coronary dominates, supplying the entire left ventricle while the right nourishes the right ventricle.

Knowledge of the blood supply to the components of the conduction system is of some help in predicting the likelihood of conduction disorders in acute myocardial infarction. The *sinus node* is supplied by a branch from the proximal right coronary artery in 55% of individuals. In the remaining 45%, the sinus node receives its blood supply from a branch arising from the proximal left circumflex artery. Involvement of these branches may lead to a "sick sinus node." The *A-V node* is supplied in 90% of cases by a branch from the distal right coronary artery, while the left circumflex supplies the A-V node in the remaining 10%. An inferior or "posterior" myocardial infarction is often due to occlusion of the right coronary artery. Consequently, disturbances in A-V node conduction are common in these infarctions.

The clinical manifestations of coronary artery narrowing or occlusion are variable. There may be:

1. No symptoms
2. Angina pectoris
3. Sudden death
4. Myocardial infarction

No symptoms occur if *collateral* or "detour" circulation is adequate for supplying the demands of the myocardium. Disease may be manifest only as nonspecific electrocardiographic changes or subtle changes in cardiac function. The supply may be adequate at rest, with changes appearing only with studies such as exercise testing or radioactive isotope scanning.

Angina pectoris is a symptom described as brief retrosternal discomfort which often radiates to the arms, jaw, or back. Angina usually is brought on by exertion or excitement, factors which increase the work of the heart and cause a discrepancy between the amount of coronary flow which is needed and the amount which can be supplied through diseased arteries. Angina does not produce myocardial damage.

Coronary occlusion causes *sudden death* in many patients, often before they can receive medical attention. Many people with angina pectoris or myocardial infarction have occlusions of several arteries, often without prior symptoms. Not until the "last straw" does the trouble develop. The heart muscle may be normal when examined grossly and with the microscope. Death has occurred so suddenly from electrical failure (arrhythmia) that infarction (tissue injury) has not yet developed. Cases of sudden death also occur in patients with coronary artery disease without a new occlusion.

Myocardial infarction describes the injury of a portion of the heart muscle when coronary artery disease has produced a severe deficiency of myocardial blood flow. Although infarction may occur without symptoms, commonly there is severe and prolonged discomfort somewhere in the front portion of the upper half of the body. Fear, sweating, nausea, or syncope often accompany it. Angina pectoris may be distinguished from myocardial infarction on a clinical basis. Angina is precipitated by exertion and relieved by rest, has a duration of less than 5 to 10 minutes, is relieved by nitroglycerin, and is not associated with laboratory or ECG signs of acute myocardial damage.

Patients with unstable angina (also called preinfarction angina, coronary insufficiency, and crescendo angina) are usually admitted to the coronary care unit. These patients have recurring chest pain, often at rest and without precipitating factors, with episodes lasting 30 or more minutes. Diagnosis depends on development of characteristic ST-T abnormalities on the electrocardiogram during episodes of pain and absence of serum enzyme abnormalities which indicate myocardial necrosis. Many patients will respond to medical therapy, chiefly nitrates and propranolol (Inderal) but some may require cardiac catheterization with coronary artery angiograms and coronary artery-vein bypass surgery.

Myocardial infarction may be associated with fever, leukocytosis, electrocardiographic changes of myocardial damage, and elevation of the serum concentration of muscle enzymes. With myocardial cell damage, these enzymes are released into the circulation. A particular enzyme is not specific for myocardial damage since enzymes are present in other tissues such as liver and brain. Creatinine-phosphokinase (CPK), serum glutamic oxaloacetic transaminase (SGOT), and lactic dehydrogenase (LDH) are enzyme determinations commonly used to confirm myocardial damage and estimate its extent. CPK rises in the early hours of myocardial infarction, reaches its peak in 24 to 36 hours and remains elevated 3 to 4 days. SGOT begins to rise somewhat later, reaching its peak in 2 to 3 days and falls to normal in 3 to 5 days. Lactic dehydrogenase rises about the same time as SGOT, peaks a little later, and remains elevated a few days longer than SGOT. This prolonged elevation is sometimes useful in detecting myocardial damage after other serum enzymes have returned to normal. See Chapter 3 for further discussion on the diagnosis of myocardial infarction.

QUESTIONS—CHAPTER 1

Fill in the appropriate choice or missing words:

1.	Disturbance in conduction is more likely to occur with occlusion of the _____ coronary artery. Such occlusions usually involve the _____ aspect of the heart.	*right* *posterior (or inferior)*
2.	Four factors which predispose to the development of coronary atherosclerosis are: A. _____ B. _____ C. _____ D. _____	*Obesity* *Hypertension* *Diabetes* *High serum cholesterol* *Cigarette smoking* *Too little exercise* *Heredity*
3.	Brief chest pain induced by exertion or excitement without acute muscle damage describes_____ .	*angina pectoris*
4.	Prolonged chest pain with subsequent evidence of heart muscle damage describes_____ .	*myocardial infarction*

5. Which characteristics are typical of angina pectoris?

    A ____ Fever, leukocytosis, and heart muscle necrosis.

    B ____ Onset with rest.

    C ____ Duration of 5–10 minutes.   *C*

    D ____ Relief with nitroglycerin.   *D*

    E ____ Discomfort in nipple area.

    F ____ Sweating, fall in blood pressure, mental confusion.

    G ____ Discomfort deep beneath the sternum.   *G*

    H ____ No histologic change in heart muscle.   *H*

    I ____ Onset with exertion.   *I*

6. The presence of cardiovascular complications such as shock or congestive heart failure.

    A ____ Increases the mortality rate in myocardial infarction.   *A*

    B ____ Increases the need for intensive coronary care.   *B*

    C ____ Is of little importance in the prognosis.

7. Two goals of the coronary care unit are:

   A. _____

   _____

   B. _____

   _____

A. *Prompt recognition and treatment of minor arrhythmias (prevention of catastrophic arrhythmias).*

B. *Preservation of viable myocardium. (reduction of myocardial work and oxygen consumption).*

8. Patients with *unstable angina* differ from those with angina pectoris because anginal pain:

   A. _____

   _____

   B. _____

   _____

A. *Is of longer duration (30 or more minutes).*

B. *Often occurs at rest and without other precipitating factors.*

SUGGESTED READING—CHAPTER 1

1. Hurst, J. W., et al: *The Heart,* Fourth Edition. McGraw-Hill, New York, 1978.

2. Spain, D. M.: Atherosclerosis. *Scientific American, 215,* 49, 1966.

3. Toronto, A. F.: *Structure and Function of the Heart.* D. C. Heath and Co., Boston, 1964.

4. Meltzer, L. E. and Dunning, A. J.: *Textbook of Coronary Care.* The Charles Press, Philadelphia, 1972.

5. Killip, T. and Kimball, J. T.: Treatment of myocardial infarction in a coronary care unit. *Amer. J. Cardiol., 20,* 457, 1967.

6. Pantridge, J. F. and Geddes, J. S.: A mobile intensive care unit in the management of myocardial infarction. *Lancet, II,* 271, 1967.

7. Grace, W. J.: *Coronary Care: Prehospital Care of Acute Myocardial Infarction.* American Heart Association, New York and Dallas, 1973.

8. Alpert, J. S. and Frances, G. S.: *Manual of Coronary Care.* Little, Brown and Co., Boston, 1977.

9. Lown, B.: Sudden cardiac death: The major challenge confronting contemporary cardiology. *Amer. J. Cardiol. 43,* 313, 1979.

10. Oliva, P. B. and Breckinridge, J. C.: Acute myocardial infarction with normal and near normal coronary arteries. *Amer. J. Cardiol., 40,* 1000, 1977.

11. Pantridge, J. F. and Adgey, A. A. J.: Prehospital care of the coronary attack. *Practical Cardiol., 5,* 56, 1979.

2

The coronary care unit

Serious arrhythmias following myocardial infarction frequently occur in the first hours after the infarction. In fact, many victims do not reach the hospital because fatal arrhythmias ensue before the patient is aware of his danger. Prompt admission to the coronary care unit is mandatory for all patients suspected of acute myocardial infarction, and certainly patients should be admitted to confirm or rule out suspected infarction.

EMERGENCY ROOM THERAPY

Patients with chest pain are often seen in the emergency room, and initial therapy is initiated there. This therapy includes:

A. A *stable I.V.,* usually with a plastic catheter, with infusion of 5% glucose/water at a slow rate.
B. *Oxygen* by nasal cannula at 4 liters per minute.
C. *Monitor* the cardiac rhythm and rate. (See Chapter 5 for various lead systems.)
D. *Treat pain*—Morphine 5 mg. I.V. or Demerol 37.5 mg. I.V.
E. *Arrhythmia prophylaxis* is often initiated with a bolus of 75–100 mg. of Lidocaine I.V. (1 mg./kg.), repeat in 10 minutes, with blood level maintained with I.V. drip at 2.0 mg./min.

STANDARDS OF TREATMENT

Few hospital staffs wish to dictate the details of care of infarction patients. However, to provide adequate care and to provide legal protection for the nurse, the order sheet must contain a considerable amount of material and be signed by the physician. For instance, the nurse must be authorized to initiate cardiopulmonary resuscitation and precordial shock. The nurse must be authorized to give certain drugs intravenously if the situation requires it and if the physician is not immediately available.

For this reason, many hospitals use a printed "Outline for Admission and Standing Orders" to spare the labor of lengthy writing for each admission. The outline is not intended to imply that each patient should be treated in the same way, but simply makes it easy for the physician to initiate care, perhaps by telephone. The patient then has benefit of a written plan of action in the event of certain complications.

OUTLINE FOR ADMISSION AND STANDING ORDERS
INTENSIVE CORONARY CARE FACILITY

Consultations: Consultations are advisable when the diagnosis remains in doubt, especially in the critically ill patient.

1. Monitor.
2. Follow standing orders for VPC's, supraventricular tachycardia and sinus or nodal bradycardia, A-V block, ventricular fibrillation, standstill. (See No. 11.)
3. Notify physician for:
   a. VPC's which are not controlled readily by drugs, especially those which are multifocal or paired
   b. Frequent APC's
   c. Significant tachycardia or bradycardia
   d. Appearance of or progression to 2nd degree or higher A-V block
   e. Other major arrhythmias
4. Start with IV with plastic cannula, 500cc.D5W to run to keep open (TKO).
5. *Oxygen*
   a. _____ 02 per nasal cannula at 4 liters per minute.
   b. _____ 02 per nasal cannula at 4 liters per minute PRN.
   c. _____ Obtain baseline arterial blood gases.
6. *Medications*
   For pain give:
   _____ Morphine 5 mg. I.V. May give additional 2 mg. I.V. every 10 minutes PRN to total 15 mg., if respiration above 12/min., ventricular rate above 60, and A-V conduction is normal.
   _____ Demerol 37.5 mg. I.V. May give additional 25 mg. I.V. every 10 minutes PRN to total 150 mg., if respirations are above 12/min., ventricular rate above 60 and A-V conduction is normal.
   _____ Lidocaine, prophylactic: Loading dose, 100 mg., given over 2 minutes, repeat in 10 minutes, or 20 mg./min. infused over 10 minutes, then continuous drip, 2–4 mg./min. for 24–30 hours.
   For daytime sedation give: _____
   For sleep at HS give: _____
   Stool softener: _____
   _____ For lesser pain, Tylenol® gr. 5-Tabs II
7. *Activity*
   a. _____ bed rest
   b. _____ bedside commode
   c. _____ stand to void
   d. _____ other _____

8. *Laboratory Tests:*
   a. ____ CPK and SGOT on admission and daily ×3.
   b. ____ EKG on admission and daily ×3.
   c. ____ Creatinine.
   d. ____ Serum potassium.
   e. ____ CPK 2 if CPK elevated.
   f. ____ Portable chest x-ray.

9. *Diet:*
   a. ____ AHA diet—2 gm. Na, low cholesterol, low fat, high polyunsaturated fat.
   b. ____ 1000 cal., 2 gm. Na, low saturated fat, full liquid × 24 hrs. Then advance to soft as tolerated.
   c. ____ Nurse may advance diet as tolerated.

10. *Vital Signs:*

    Take q 4 hours. Omit 2400 and 0400 if stable ____ . Notify physician if BP below ____ mg./Hg.

11. *Treatment of Arrhythmias:*
    a. Ventricular fibrillation: Follow standing orders.
    b. Ventricular standstill: Follow standing orders.
    c. Ventricular premature beats ("Class B").
       If more than 6 per minute, *or*
       If more than 10% of cycles are VPC's, *or*
       If multifocal, *or*
       If paired, *or*
       If steadily becoming more frequent:
       (1) If on prophylactic drip, lidocaine, 70 mg. (1 mg./kg.) I.V. over 2 minutes, repeat after 4 minutes if not effective, and notify physician.
       (2) If not on prophylactic drip:
           (a) Loading dose, 100 mg. given over 2 minutes, start on continuous drip, 2–4 mg./min., repeat bolus of 100 mg. in 10 minutes.
           (b) If not effective, give additional lidocaine, 50–100 mg. I.V. over 2 minutes and notify physician.
           (c) Reduce doses by 50% in patients with congestive heart failure, shock, or liver disease, or who are over 70 years old.
    d. Ventricular tachycardia or flutter
       (1) Brief paroxysms: Treat as "Class B" VPC's.
       (2) Sustained, but without cardiovascular collapse: Treat as "Class B" VPC's.
       (3) Sustained, with cardiovascular collapse:
           (a) Precordial shock, 200 W.S.
           (b) If effective, follow with lidocaine drip, 2–4 mg./min.
           (c) If not effective, give lidocaine, 70 mg. (1 mg./kg.) I.V. push, and repeat precordial shock, 300 W.S.
           (d) If effective, follow with lidocaine drip, 2–4 mg./min.
           (e) Notify physician.

   e. Sinus or nodal bradycardia
- (1) Rate of 50–60, BP and mental status satisfactory, skin warm and dry: notify physician.
- (2) Rate 50–60 with fall in BP, confusion or stupor, cool or sweaty skin: Give atropine 0.5 mg. I.V. and notify physician.
- (3) Rate 48 or below: Give atropine 0.5 mg. I.V. and notify physician.

   f. A-V Block, first degree: notify physician.

   g. A-V block, second degree:
- (1) Atropine—0.5 mg. I.V. and notify physician.
- (2) If no response in 3 minutes, start Isuprel® drip (0.4 mg. in 500 cc. 5% G/W) at 20 drips per minute unless VPC's develop. Notify physician.

   h. A-V block, complete:
- (1) Start Isuprel® drip as above.

THE CCU AND THE NURSE

Patients admitted to the CCU exhibit various degrees of anxiety. Since anxiety increases cardiac work and may also be a factor in producing serious arrhythmias, steps should be taken to reduce anxiety wherever possible. Reassurance and confidence should be reflected by the staff and the surroundings. The coronary care unit should be an area which is comfortable, spacious and quiet. Contact with the outside world such as newspapers, visitors and music should be permitted when appropriate to the patient's condition. A calendar and a clock are important to the patient's orientation.

There are few places in the hospital where the patient's welfare is so dependent on the nurse as in the CCU. Important characteristics of the CCU nurse include the following:

1. Be well trained in a formal training program.
2. Present an air of confidence and control to the patient.
3. Explain procedures to the patient and family to allay anxiety.
4. Provide important initial rehabilitation of the patient. (See Chapter 14.)

DIET IN THE CORONARY CARE UNIT

In general, diet is determined by the clinical status of the patient. After arrival in the CCU, the patient should not be fed for several hours until his or her clinical state is stable and initial therapy has been instituted. To reduce postprandial myocardial work, early diets are generally low in calories and salt. A 1000-calorie, 2 gm. sodium, full liquid diet is often prescribed the first two days. To limit cardiac work, it is preferable to serve six small feedings. For some patients, sodium restriction may not be necessary. If the clinical status indicates, the patient may advance to a solid, bland diet in succeeding days, and a low-saturated fat diet should be introduced early. Dietary therapy of specific problems should also be started: calorie reduction for obesity, and sodium restriction for hypertension.

Constipation resulting in straining at stool should be avoided by adding a bulk laxative and a stool softener.

SUGGESTED READING—CHAPTER 2

1. Cassem, N. H., Hackett, T. P., Bascom, C. and Wishnea, H. A.: Reactions of coronary patients to the CCU nurse. *Amer. J. Nurs., 70,* 319, 1970.

2. Grace, W. J. and Keyloun, V.: *The Coronary Care Unit.* Appleton Century Crofts, New York, 1970.

3. Hemzacek, K. I.: Dietary protocol for the patient who has suffered a myocardial infarction. *J. Amer. Dietetic Assn., 72,* 182, 1978.

4. Burch, G. E.: Sick people's food. *Amer. Heart J., 85,* 279, 1973.

5. Gazes, P. C. and Gaddy, J. E.: Bedside management of acute myocardial infarction. *Amer. Heart J., 97,* 782, 1979.

6. Harrison, D. C.: Should lidocaine be administered routinely to all patients after acute myocardial infarction? *Circulation, 58,* 581, 1978.

3

Common tests in myocardial infarction

ELECTROCARDIOGRAM

The electrocardiogram is the standard in the diagnosis of myocardial infarction. Classic *transmural myocardial infarction* produces Q waves in leads which reflect anatomical regions.

> Anterior leads—I, AVL, V1–V6
> Lateral leads—I, AVL, V4–V6
> Inferior and posterior leads—II, III, AVF

In acute infarction, ST elevation and T wave inversion are associated with the Q waves, and change in serial tracings.

Non-transmural infarction is associated with similar ST-T changes without Q waves.

However, ST-T changes and even Q waves can occur at times in the absence of myocardial infarction.

ENZYMES

The elevation of enzymes in the serum is helpful in diagnosing and estimating the extent of myocardial infarction. The enzymes are released into the circulation with myocardial cell damage.

Creatinine phosphokinase (CPK), serum glutamic oxaloacetic transaminase (SGOT), and lactic dehydrogenase (LDH) are the enzyme determinations commonly used. Since these enzymes occur in other tissues besides the myocardium, their elevation may be non-specific. This has led to the development of isoenzymes such as CPK2 which are more specific for myocardium.

Serum enzymes and isoenzymes are most helpful in the diagnosis or exclusion of small myocardial infarction associated with nonspecific ECG abnormalities or when myocardial infarction is masked by left bundle branch block. They are also helpful in monitoring extension of infarction or "re-infarction." Large infarctions do not require enzymes for diagnosis but the level may reflect the extent of myocardial damage. On the other hand, enzyme levels in the serum are related to the rate of release and rate of clearance, so that some patients with large infarctions may not show high levels.

FEATURES OF SERUM ENZYMES

Enzyme	Onset	Peak	Return to Normal
CPK	6–12 hr.	24 hr.	3–4 days
SGOT	8–12 hr.	18–36 hr.	3–4 days
LDH	24–48 hr.	3–6 days	7–14 days

Elevation of CPK occurs most rapidly, while elevation of LDH is more delayed. This may be helpful in detecting myocardial infarction when there has been a delay in the patient being seen.

CPK may be elevated in pulmonary infarction, after intramuscular injection, exercise, tachycardia, coronary arteriograms, seizures, and hyperthyroidism.

SGOT may be elevated in liver disease, congestive heart failure, shock, and skeletal muscle diseases.

LDH may be increased in congestive heart failure, shock, pulmonary embolus, myocarditis, cardioversion, neoplasm, and hemolysis. These nonspecific elevations have led to the development of serum isoenzymes of CPK and LDH which are more specific for myocardial damage. CPK2 (M-B fraction) is very specific for myocardial damage, peaking at about 18 hours, with significantly lower levels at 12 and 24 hours. It may return to normal by 36 hours. Absence of elevations of CPK2 during this period virtually excludes the diagnosis of acute myocardial infarction, and the patient may be transferred to a less costly area or discharged if the clinical situation does not warrant further study. The "myocardial" LDH isoenzyme is less specific and may be elevated in hemolysis and pulmonary infarction.

ARTERIAL BLOOD GASES

Acute myocardial infarction is often associated with hypoxia because of increased stiffness of the lungs related to elevated left ventricular filling pressure or low cardiac output. Chronic pulmonary disease may also be present.

Since arterial hypoxia may aggravate myocardial ischemia, supplemental oxygen administration at 2–4 L./min. usually is used. Arterial blood gases are helpful in determining the rate and method (nasal prongs, face mask) of oxygen delivery.

CHEST X-RAY

Chest x-rays during the first 3 days after infarction are often helpful in detecting elevated left ventricular filling pressure, elevated pulmonary capillary pressure, and "pulmonary vascular congestion." These early signs of left ventricular failure may appear before other clinical signs such as dyspnea and rales. X-ray changes may persist even after adequate therapy. Insertion of a flow-directed catheter to measure pulmonary capillary wedge pressure and pulmonary artery oxygen saturation may be helpful in the further management of the patient. (See Chapter 4.)

SUGGESTED READING — CHAPTER 3

1. Horan, L. G., Flowers, N. C. and Johnson, J. C.: Significance of the diagnostic Q wave of myocardial infarction. *Circulation, 43,* 428, 1971.

2. Sobel, B. E. and Shell, W. E.: Serum enzyme determinations in the diagnosis and assessment of myocardial infarction. (Symposium on Myocardial Infarction, 1972, Part 2.) *Circulation, 45,* 471, 1972.

3. Kostuk, W., Barr, J. W., Simon, A. L. and Ross, J., Jr.: Correlations between the chest film and hemodynamics in acute myocardial infarction. *Circulation, 48,* 624, 1973.

4. Fillmore, S. J., Shapiro, M. and Killip, T.: Arterial oxygen tension in acute myocardial infarction. Serial analysis of clinical state and blood gas changes. *Amer. Heart J., 79,* 620, 1970.

4

Physiology of abnormal rhythms, shock, and congestive failure

---
CARDIAC OUTPUT

Cardiac output represents the amount of blood pumped by the heart each minute.

Cardiac output is determined by the *heart rate* and *stroke volume* (the volume of blood pumped with each beat) and may be expressed mathematically as:

$$CO = HR \times SV$$

Cardiac Output equals *Heart Rate* times *Stroke Volume*

Cardiac reserve represents the potential increase in cardiac output over the resting cardiac output which the heart can produce on demand.

Cardiac output may be altered by changing:

A. HEART RATE
B. STROKE VOLUME

Cardiac reserve is diminished by myocardial disease which limits heart rate or stroke volume.

A. Heart Rate

1. *Tachycardia.* Normally, the heart rate may double or triple to increase cardiac output. The heart ejects during systole and fills during diastole. The duration of systole changes little as the heart rate increases, while diastole shortens greatly. *Tachycardia results in less time for the heart to fill between each contraction.*

Study the graph below:

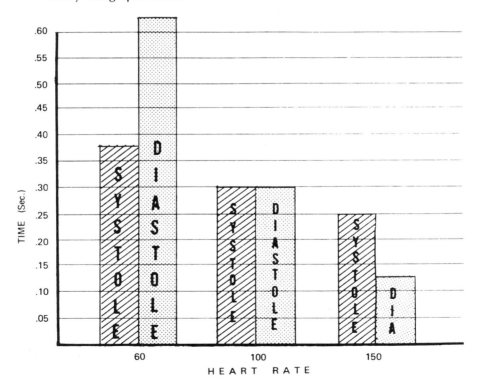

As the heart rate increases from 60 to 150, notice that systole shortens only slightly while diastole is greatly shortened.

> An excessively rapid heart rate may shorten diastole so much that decreased filling results in decreased stroke volume and thus decreased cardiac output.

Coronary artery blood flow is determined by the aortic blood pressure, cardiac output, and heart rate. The coronary arteries are squeezed during ventricular contraction (systole). Therefore, *coronary blood flow* occurs largely during diastole.

> Extreme shortening of diastole results in a fall in coronary blood flow.

Reduction of cardiac output and coronary blood flow with increased cardiac work produced by tachycardia may lead to angina, arrhythmias, further infarction, congestive heart failure, or shock.

2. *Bradycardia.* At normal heart rates, most of the ventricular filling occurs during the first two-thirds of diastole. Further lengthening of diastole does not lead to additional filling of the heart. If the rate is too slow, the product, Heart Rate × Stroke Volume, is low. This is especially true in myocardial infarction since stroke volume is often low. The resulting low aortic pressure and cardiac output lead to low coronary and tissue blood flow.

> Low HR × Low SV = Low CO

Poor *cerebral* blood flow may result in mental confusion or syncope (Adams-Stokes attacks). Poor *coronary* blood flow may result in angina, arrhythmias, further infarction, congestive heart failure, or shock. Poor *renal* blood flow may result in oliguria, sodium retention, and subsequent congestive heart failure. Poor *peripheral* flow results in cool, cyanotic extremities.

Blood returning to the heart in the venous system may "back up" under higher pressure if not pumped away by the heart. Both bradycardia and tachycardia may result in an increase in venous pressure, both systemic and pulmonic.

Tachycardia and bradycardia may produce:

1. Fall in cardiac output.
2. Fall in blood pressure.
3. Fall in coronary blood flow.
4. Fall in splanchnic, renal, and cerebral blood flow.
5. Increased venous pressure.
6. Increased cardiac work.

B. Stroke Volume

Stroke volume, the other determinant of cardiac output, does not change much with usual activities in the normal individual, but may double with extreme exertion.

Stroke volume increases by two mechanisms:

1. More complete emptying of the ventricle, resulting in less blood remaining in the heart at the end of systole. Physiologists call this the *end-systolic residue*.
2. Increased filling of the heart during diastole, resulting in a stretching of the myocardial fibers. Physiologists call this the *end-diastolic volume*.

Stroke volume may be increased by:

1. *More complete emptying* during systole (decreased end-systolic residue).
2. *Greater filling* during diastole (increased end-diastolic volume).

The *end-diastolic volume* has another significant role in heart muscle performance. Myocardial fibers, lengthened by a greater diastolic volume, respond with a greater force of systolic contraction. However, this is true only to a certain amount of filling; beyond this, excessive stretching results in a weaker contraction. At this point, "heart failure" is said to be present. This fundamental principle of heart muscle behavior was described by Starling and has been called *The Law of the Heart*.

THE LAW OF THE HEART

Within physiologic limits, a larger end-diastolic volume results in a greater strength of systolic contraction.

The graph below illustrates the principle:

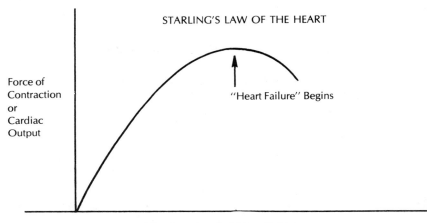

STARLING'S LAW OF THE HEART

Force of Contraction or Cardiac Output

"Heart Failure" Begins

Fiber Length or End-Diastolic Volume

Acute myocardial infarction usually causes a reduced stroke volume. The normal contractile state and efficiency are impaired by the infarction.

The patient with an acute myocardial infarction not only has a reduced stroke volume but is *unable to increase the stroke volume* for additional demands; the stroke volume is "fixed" at a low level.

$$CO = HR \times SV$$

An increased rate is the remaining mechanism for increasing the cardiac output.

Excessive tachycardia or bradycardia reduces cardiac output. The precise rate limits, beyond which there is a fall in cardiac output, depend upon the degree of myocardial damage and the degree to which stroke volume is fixed. Heart rates above 120 or below 50/min. usually adversely affect the patient with acute infarction.

OTHER CAUSES OF FALL IN CARDIAC OUTPUT IN ARRHYTHMIAS

A. Uncoordinated Contraction

Normally, systole proceeds in a coordinated manner, so that the squeezing action of the ventricles produces the most effective emptying. Arrhythmias arising in the ventricles produce a different pattern of contraction, just as they produce a different QRS pattern on the ECG. With such a contraction, poorer emptying of the ventricles occurs.

An increase in heart rate to 150/min. by sinus tachycardia may increase cardiac output and coronary blood flow. Ventricular tachycardia at the same rate may reduce cardiac output and coronary blood flow because of uncoordinated contraction.

B. Loss of Atrial Kick

Proper time relationships between atrial and ventricular contractions contribute to a normal stroke volume. Under ordinary circumstances, atrial systole occurs at the very end of ventricular filling, distending the ventricles with a final load of blood. The ventricles, thus distended, are stimulated to contract more efficiently. Stroke volume ordinarily is maximum when atrial contraction occurs 0.12 to 0.20 seconds before ventricular contraction. In *atrial fibrillation,* the atria do not contribute to ventricular filling, and cardiac output often is reduced, even when the ventricular rate is not excessive.

A-V dissociation, heart block, nodal rhythm and ventricular premature contractions are other situations in which the ventricles are not filled optimally by a properly timed atrial contraction.

C.   Nonuniform Ventricular Filling Period

Atrial fibrillation often is associated with considerable irregularity of rhythm. Although the *average* ventricular rate may be normal, this average is made up of short and long cycles, neither of which is optimal.

The premature beat comes early in diastole, before complete diastolic filling has occurred. *Thus a premature beat usually is associated with a reduced stroke volume,* even though it uses almost as much energy as an effective beat. In your next patient, note the weak pulse associated with premature beats. Although a premature contraction may be *heard* with the stethoscope over the apex, it may not be *felt* with your fingers on the radial artery. This is the origin of the pulse deficit, discerned by simultaneously counting the apical and radial rate.

SOME CAUSES OF LOW CARDIAC OUTPUT

	Heart Rate		*Stroke Volume*		*Cardiac Output*	*Mechanism*
	Too fast		Low		Low	Short diastolic filling time
Example:	180/min.	×	20 ml.	=	3.6 L.	
	Normal		Low		Low	Poor contraction
Example:	80/min.	×	45 ml.	=	3.6 L.	
	Too slow		Normal		Low	Limited by slow rate
Example:	40/min.	×	90 ml.	=	3.6 L.	

COMPENSATORY MECHANISMS WHEN CARDIAC OUTPUT IS LOW

When cardiac output is low, compensatory mechanisms may assist vital tissues as discussed below.

A.   Increased Oxygen Extraction

The *body tissues* extract only a portion of the oxygen present in arterial blood. When blood flow is reduced, many tissues are able to compensate by extracting more of the available oxygen. *Heart muscle,* however, cannot use this means to compensate for low coronary flow; even with normal flow, oxygen extraction is nearly maximal.

B. Redistribution of Blood Flow

Small arterial vessels may alter their size by neural and humoral control. Dilation of the vessels results in more flow to the tissue, while constriction produces less flow. When cardiac output is limited, constriction of the vessels to the skin, muscles, kidneys, and other abdominal organs may shunt blood to more vital organs such as the heart and brain.

Such a compensatory mechanism is useful for only a limited period since serious metabolic changes may occur in tissues deprived of adequate blood flow. It is these metabolic changes which account for many of the derangements in severe or irreversible shock. Vasopressor therapy in shock is of limited value because it accentuates preexisting, harmful vasoconstriction.

C. Increased Blood Volume and Venous Return

A fall in cardiac output causes diminished renal blood flow and retention of sodium and water. Blood volume is increased. Venous return is augmented and cardiac output may increase. (See "The Law of the Heart" in this chapter.)

D. Good Nursing Care

Starling did not mention it, but skillful nursing provides additional help when cardiac output is low.

Many nursing measures are designed to reduce oxygen requirements so that a lowered flow is adequate for body needs. Rest, relief of pain, a tranquil environment, and the tranquility of spirit which derives from an awareness that the care is excellent—each of these may be needed to survive a period of low cardiac output.

CONGESTIVE HEART FAILURE

Congestive heart failure is a term used to describe clinical syndromes with congestion of blood in the lungs (left ventricular failure) or congestion of blood in the liver and peripheral veins (right heart failure).

Two useful concepts have been postulated to explain the development of the symptoms of congestive heart failure:

A.   **"Backward failure"** supposes that one ventricle, at normal filling pressure, is unable to expel the volume of blood pumped to it by the stronger ventricle. This produces high venous pressure and congestion behind the failing ventricle. (Review Starling's Law of the Heart, page 26.)

Example No. 1:   Left ventricle fails. Blood backs up in the pulmonary veins and capillaries. Congestion stiffens lung tissue, producing dyspnea. Fluid leaks into alveoli, producing rales and frothy sputum.

Example No. 2:   Right ventricle fails. Blood backs up in the vena cavae, producing distended neck veins, enlargement of the liver, ascites, and peripheral edema.

B.   **"Forward failure"** assumes that the primary problem is inadequate blood flow to the kidneys. Sodium and water retention result. Blood volume increases, causing increased venous pressure, pulmonary congestion, hepatic congestion, edema, and weight gain.

Most congestive heart failure is a combination of the processes in "forward" and "backward" failure.

Mechanism of Signs and Symptoms

As the ventricle weakens, it may need greater diastolic filling to achieve the required force of contraction:

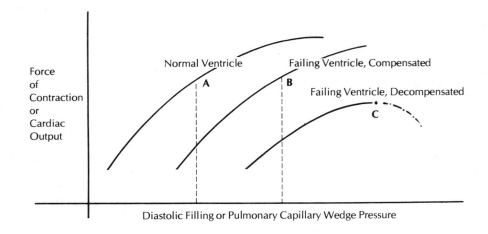

In the graph on page 30, note the additional diastolic filling required by the failing ventricle (point B) to achieve the same force of contraction as the normal ventricle (point A).

A failing left ventricle will need increased diastolic filling to pump its usual volume of blood. This increase is reflected in a higher pressure in the left atrium and the pulmonary veins.

Eventually the patient may "decompensate" with:

1. *Inadequate pumping.* Note that diastolic filling at point C, with maximum force of contraction, is less than at points A and B.

2. *High venous pressure.* Note the large diastolic volume required to produce the maximum force of contraction (point C). High venous pressure stiffens the lungs producing dyspnea and cough. Fluid leaking into the alveoli results in further dyspnea, cough, rales, and reduced oxygen exchange.

Inadequate pumping may develop gradually, producing fluid retention and congestive heart failure. Or it may develop with dramatic suddenness, producing acute pulmonary edema or cardiogenic shock.

PULMONARY ARTERY DIASTOLIC AND PULMONARY WEDGE PRESSURES

Left ventricular filling pressure is a good index of left ventricular function. Left ventricular decompensation, particularly when acute as in myocardial infarction, may not correlate well with central venous pressure. In such situations, left ventricular filling pressure may be quite high when central venous pressure is either normal or only slightly elevated, and volume loading may be hazardous. Flow-directed balloon catheters (Swan-Ganz) have been used to obtain pulmonary artery pressures or pulmonary "capillary wedge" pressures. The catheter, similar to that used for obtaining central venous pressure, is advanced to the right atrium. At this point, a small balloon on the tip is inflated with air. This balloon allows the blood flow to carry it into the right ventricle and out into the pulmonary artery without the use of fluoroscopy. Pulmonary artery pressure then can be continuously monitored by use of a strain gauge. In the absence of chronic obstructive pulmonary disease or mitral stenosis, the pulmonary artery diastolic pressure correlates well with the left ventricular diastolic pressure. The catheter may be advanced to a small pulmonary artery branch, the balloon inflated to briefly occlude the vessel, and pulmonary capillary wedge pressure obtained. This pressure is identical with left atrial pressure, and in the absence of mitral valve lesions, is similar to the filling pressure of the left ventricle.

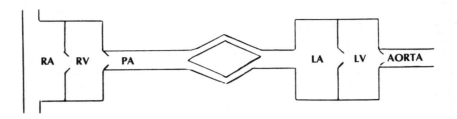

Note in the diagram above that there are no valves between the pulmonary artery and the left atrium. The pulmonary artery diastolic pressure will be similar to the left atrial pressure.

Normal Values

Pulmonary diastolic pressure is normally between 4 and 13 mm. Hg. (average 9 mm. Hg.). Pulmonary capillary wedge pressure is normally 5 to 13 mm. Hg. Elevation of pulmonary artery diastolic pressure (in the absence of chronic pulmonary disease) or pulmonary wedge pressure indicates elevated left atrial pressure. This, in turn, indicates elevated left ventricular filling pressure and left ventricular decompensation (in the absence of mitral valve disease).

BLOOD PRESSURE CONTROL

Pressure receptors, present in the aortic arch and carotid arteries, send signals to the brain, which responds by signaling the heart and peripheral blood vessels. If the pressure is too low, the heart rate increases and peripheral blood vessels constrict. If the pressure is too high, the heart rate slows and peripheral vessels dilate. Many other complex mechanisms, not discussed here, also are important in maintaining blood pressure. This control system does help recall some of the signs we recognize as shock, such as tachycardia and pale, cool skin.

It is important to recognize that cuff pressures do not accurately record arterial pressure, especially with severe vasoconstriction. When low cuff pressures occur, measurement of arterial pressure by direct cannulation of the radial, brachial, or femoral artery may be indicated. Accurate pressure readings may be obtained also with a Doppler flow meter.

Cardiogenic shock is a clinical syndrome resulting from inadequate blood flow to vital organs because of a profound fall in cardiac output.

Shock in myocardial infarction is usually due to decreased cardiac output secondary to myocardial injury and inadequate pumping.

When cardiac output is low, constriction of blood vessels in the skin, muscle, gut, and kidney shunts the available blood flow to the heart and brain. The pale, cool, sweaty skin commonly seen in shock is due to shunting of blood, a sign of inadequate cardiac output. Oliguria results from decreased renal blood flow. If these compensatory measures are not sufficient to provide adequate blood flow to the brain and the heart, confusion, restlessness, coma, and arrhythmias may result. If compensatory mechanisms are not sufficient, tissue perfusion is inadequate, cellular function is impaired, metabolic derangements are severe, and shock may be irreversible.

A low blood volume secondary to dehydration may contribute to impaired cardiac output, and thus to the development of shock. During the early infarction period, patients may eat and drink little. Vomiting, sweating, and fever may increase fluid loss. Significant dehydration may result if these fluid losses are not replaced.

Measurement of pulmonary artery diastolic pressure and pulmonary capillary wedge pressure are used to evaluate adequacy of diastolic filling pressure. A low pulmonary artery capillary wedge pressure or pulmonary diastolic pressure in a patient with shock suggests that blood volume may be increased safely and profitably to augment cardiac filling and cardiac output. A high pulmonary capillary wedge pressure or pulmonary diastolic pressure in a patient with shock suggests that pump failure is a major factor and that further increase in blood volume will be hazardous.

BLOOD GASES AND pH

The gases, oxygen and carbon dioxide, are always present in the body, the former used as fuel in the production of energy, the latter as an end product of this process. In a mixture of gases, each exerts a pressure in relation to its own concentration. The concentration of these gases is also related to their concentration in the alveoli of the lungs and the perfusion of the lung capillaries by the blood. Measurement of these gases in arterial blood gives an index of pulmonary ventilation and perfusion and may be helpful in assessing cardiac function and the result of therapeutic interventions, particularly in the treatment of shock. *The measurement of the oxygen content in mixed venous blood, as obtained from the pulmonary artery, may give additional data reflecting peripheral metabolism, and as an index of cardiac output.* A low pulmonary artery oxygen saturation suggests increased peripheral oxygen extraction due to a low cardiac output.

All body fluids, with the exception of gastric juice, are mildly acid or alkaline. The amount of acidity or alkalinity is dependent on the concentration of hydrogen ions, and is indicated by the symbol pH. A pH of 7.4 is normal, less than 7.4 indicates acidosis, and above 7.4 alkalosis. If tissue perfusion is poor as in congestive heart failure or shock, metabolism will be carried out with an oxygen deficit, resulting in the accumulation of acids which would normally be oxidized to carbon dioxide. The end result is increasing acidity of the blood or "metabolic acidosis." Metabolic acidosis may be partially compensated by increasing pulmonary ventilation and "blowing off" carbon dioxide. Poor pulmonary ventilation may result in accumulation of carbon dioxide (respiratory acidosis), while overventilation may reduce carbon dioxide and lower acidity (respiratory alkalosis).

Normal Values

The partial pressure of oxygen (PaO_2) normally is about 100 mm. of mercury in the arterial blood and alveoli at sea level.

The partial pressure of carbon dioxide ($PaCO_2$) normally is about 40 mm. in arterial blood and alveoli at sea level.

Arterial blood has a pH of 7.35 to 7.45. The limits compatible with life are about 7.0 and 7.8.

ELECTROLYTES

The body water acts as a solvent for many substances such as sodium chloride, glucose, and urea. Electrolytes are substances which split into ions when dissolved in water. Some ions have a positive charge such as sodium and potassium and are called cations; others such as chloride and phosphate have a negative charge and are called anions. The total cations always balance the total anions. Ions are measured in milliequivalents per liter (mEq./L.). Electrolytes in the plasma may be altered in various ways such as by loss in urine, stool, or vomitus, concentration or dilution by changes in body water, or shifts in or out of the body cells. Electrolyte balance is maintained by the kidneys and lungs and hormones secreted by the pituitary, adrenal, and parathyroid glands.

Electrolyte imbalance, particularly alterations in potassium and calcium, may produce cardiac arrhythmias which may be unusually resistant to therapy with antiarrhythmic drugs. Hypoxia and alterations in acid-base balance, particularly metabolic acidosis, are also important in the production of cardiac arrhythmias.

Normal Values

The plasma electrolytes which are commonly determined clinically are:

	Normal Value
Sodium (Na+)	135–147 mEq./L.
Potassium (K+)	3.8–5.0 mEq./L.
Calcium (Ca++)	4.3–5.5 mEq./L.
Chloride (Cl−)	100–106 mEq./L.
Bicarbonate (HCO$_3$ −)	26–30 mEq./L.
Phosphate (PO$_4$ =)	1.7–2.3 mEq./L.

ILLUSTRATIVE CASES

1. The patient is receiving rapid transfusions for gastrointestinal bleeding which developed during anticoagulant therapy for myocardial infarction. The skin is cold and clammy. The pulmonary capillary wedge pressure (PCW) is 11 mm. Hg. The arterial pressure is 60 mm. Hg. Urine volume is 15 ml./hr.

    The physician's order would read:

    (1) Stop transfusion stat and order 250 ml. phlebotomy.

    (2) Continue transfusion. Record PCW every 15 minutes and report if PCW is creeping upward or exceeds 15 mm.Hg.

If you answered (1), you were wrong. A PCW of 11 mm. Hg. is not particularly low, but neither is it dangerously high. Low blood pressure and low urine volume, and the cold, clammy skin, in conjunction with the history of hemorrhage, all indicate low blood volume.

(2) is the proper answer, for therapy would be designed to steadily increase blood volume until signs of shock disappeared or the PCW advanced too far.

2. The patient was admitted to the CCU two days ago with an extensive anterior myocardial infarction. He had repeated vomiting and wretching the first day. Yesterday he had an intake of 840 cc. Temperature was 102° yesterday and is 103° today. He has not voided since last evening. Pulse is 128 per minute and blood pressure is 60/40. Skin is cool and moist. Because of hypotension, a flow-directed catheter is introduced into the pulmonary artery and a pulmonary capillary wedge pressure is obtained. Initial reading is 6 mm. Hg.

The physician's order would read:

(1) Start dopamine, 50 mg./min., then adjust to maintain systolic pressure at 100 mm. Catheterize, record urine volume every 15 minutes. Give digoxin, 1.0 mg., I.V.

(2) Give 200 cc. 5% glucose in water over 10 minute period. Notify physician if PCW rises 5 mm. Hg. or more during infusion and fails to fall with 2 mm. Hg. of original value after infusion. If no rise in PCW, give additional test dose of 200 cc. of 5% glucose in water over 10 minutes and repeat PCW readings.

If you answered (1), you were wrong. The patient has shock due to hypovolemia. Fever, vomiting, and low oral intake may result in low circulating volume and hypovolemic shock.

Administration of a challenge dose of 200 cc. of 5% glucose in water over 10 minutes without a rise in the PCW would suggest hypovolemia, and additional challenge doses could be given until the hypotension is corrected or the PCW rises.

3. The following case is illustrative of the use of pulmonary capillary wedge pressure in some cases of shock in acute myocardial infarction.

A 62-year-old printer developed mild, brief retrosternal discomfort, unrelated to activity, three weeks prior to admission. Eight hours before admission he began having severe retrosternal chest pain with dyspnea.

Hospital course:

Day 1. Admitted directly to ward. After one hour, transferred to CCU and promptly developed ventricular fibrillation, reversed by 400 W-S precordial shock. Then given 70 mg. lidocaine bolus followed by drip, 4 mg./min. ECG: Acute anterior infarction. SGOT: 40 U. Intake 100 cc. oral; 2125 cc. I.V. Output 820 cc. BP 160/100. Pulse 120.

Day 2. Dyspneic. BP 150/100. Pulse 110. Rales both bases. SGOT: 208 U. Intake 460 cc. oral; 2050 cc. I.V. Output 1600 cc. after I.V. Lasix 40 mg.

Day 3. No dyspnea. Lungs clear. BP 110/80. Pulse 120. Intake 590 cc. oral; 900 cc. I.V. Output 1880 cc.

Day 4. Pale, cool skin. No sweating. Basilar rales. BP 80/60. Pulse 120. PCW 5 mm. Hg.

Challenge doses of 200 cc. 5% G/W given I.V. as follows:

Time	Dose	PCW (mm.Hg.)	BP	Pulse	Urine Output
0 min.	200 cc.	5	80/60	120	0
20 "	200 cc.	5	90/60	120	0
40 "	200 cc.	6	110/72	110	0
60 "	200 cc.	6	114/80	100	0
80 "	200 cc.	7	120/80	90	0
100 "	200 cc.	9	116/80	84	0
120 "	200 cc.	9	120/82	90	125
140 "	200 cc.	9	120/80	80	200
24 hr.	2475 cc.	9	120/80	80	2390

Volume expanders such as dextran or saline may be used for part of the fluid challenge.

QUESTIONS—CHAPTER 4

1. The volume of blood pumped by the heart each minute is called the _____ .	*cardiac output*
2. The volume of blood expelled with each contraction of the heart is called the _____ .	*stroke volume*
3. Cardiac output is determined by the stroke volume and the: A. ____ Oxygen extraction. B. ____ Heart rate. C. ____ Blood pressure.	 *B*
4. List four signs for "right ventricular failure": A. _____ B. _____ C. _____ D. _____	 *Liver enlargement* *Ascites* *Weight gain* *Edema* *Distended neck veins*
5. The heart expels blood during _____; the heart fills during _____ .	*systole* *diastole*
6. If diastole is shortened, the heart will have less time to _____ .	*fill*

7. Tachycardia may produce a fall in cardiac output because _____

_____

_____

_____ .

decreased filling time results in a fall in stroke volume

---

8. Bradycardia allows complete filling of the heart, but a low cardiac output may result because _____

_____

_____

_____

_____

_____ .

the volume of blood pumped is limited by the slow rate, or the product of rate times stroke volume is low

---

9. Most coronary blood flow occurs during_____ .

A. _____ systole.

B. _____ diastole.

B

10. Indicate by an arrow (↑ or ↓) the effect of excessive tachycardia and bradycardia on:

    ____ A. Cardiac output.   ↓

    ____ B. Venous pressure.   ↑

    ____ C. Coronary blood flow.   ↓

    ____ D. Tissue blood flow.   ↓

    ____ E. Cardiac work.   ↑

    ____ F. Blood pressure.   ↓

---

11. The patient with a myocardial infarction alters his cardiac output by changes in heart rate because _____

    _____   *the stroke volume is low and "fixed"*

    _____

    _____ .

---

12. Cardiac output may be reduced in atrial fibrillation because of:

    A. _____   *Increased heart rate.*

    B. _____   *Loss of atrial kick.*

    C. _____   *Non-uniform ventricular filling.*

13. Cardiac output may be reduced in ventricular tachycardia because of:

A. ______________ *Rapid heart rate.*

B. ______________ *Uncoordinated contraction.*

C. ______________ *Loss of atrial kick.*

14.

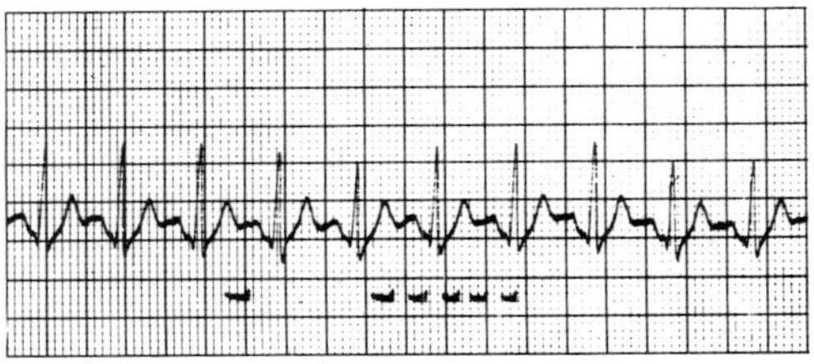

The above ECG was recorded during cardiogenic shock. What is the rhythm?

______________ *Sinus tachycardia*

This reflex tachycardia is a response to ______________ . *low cardiac output*

15.

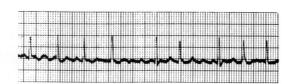

This patient developed angina and hypotension.

A. What is the arrhythmia?

_____

Atrial fibrillation

B. What would be the initial aim of treatment?

_____

Slow the heart

16.

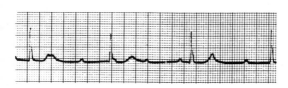

A 62-year-old male suddenly became sweaty, confused, and pale with a blood pressure of 70/32.

A. What is the arrhythmia?

_____

Third degree (complete) A-V block.

B. What would be the aim of treatment?

_____

Increase the ventricular rate.

17. Pulmonary capillary wedge pressure may be used to:

   A. ____ Indicate heart failure.

   B. ____ Indicate deficiency in blood volume.

   C. ____ Determine the method of treatment for shock.

A

B

C

---

18. Pulmonary capillary wedge pressure measures:

   A. ____ Left atrial pressure.

   B. ____ Left ventricular pressure.

   C. ____ Left ventricular filling pressure.

A

C

---

19. A high pulmonary artery pressure and pulmonary capillary wedge pressure occur in:

   A. ____ Mitral stenosis.

   B. ____ Chronic pulmonary disease.

   C. ____ Left ventricular failure.

A

C

---

20. A pulmonary capillary wedge pressure of 4 mm. Hg. in a patient with hypotension suggests:

   A. ____ Left ventricular failure.

   B. ____ Dehydration.

   C. ____ Blood loss due to hemorrhage.

B

C

SUGGESTED READING — CHAPTER 4

1. Swan, H. J. C., Ganz, W., Forrester, J., Marcus, H., Diamond, G. and Chonette, D.: Catheterization of the heart in man with the use of a flow directed balloon tipped catheter. *N. Eng. J. Med. 283,* 447, 1970.

2. Cohn, J. N.: Blood pressure measurement in shock. Mechanism of inaccuracy in auscultatory and palpatory methods. *J. Amer. Med. Assn., 199,* 972, 1967.

3. Corwin, J. H. and Moseley, T.: Subclavian venipuncture and central venous pressure: Technique and application. *Amer. Surgeon, 32,* 413, 1966.

4. Broden, M. I. and Cohn, J. N.: Evolution of abnormalities in left ventricular function after myocardial infarction. *Circulation, 46,* 731, 1972.

5. Russell, R. O., Hunt, D. and Rackley, C. E.: Left ventricular hemodynamics in anterior and inferior myocardial infarction. *Amer. J. Cardiol., 32,* 8, 1973.

6. Sonnenblick, E. H. and Skelton, C. L.: Myocardial energetics: Basic principles and clinical applications. *N. Eng. J. Med., 285,* 668, 1971.

7. Crexells, C., Chatterjee, K., Forrester, J. S., Dikshit, K., and Swan, H. J. C.: Optimal level of filling pressure in the left side of the heart in acute myocardial infarction. *N. Eng. J. Med., 289,* 1263, 1973.

8. Franciosa, J. A., Guiha, N. M., Lemas, C. J., Paz, S. and Cohn, J. N.: Arterial pressure as a determinant of left ventricular filling pressure after acute myocardial infarction. *Amer. J. Cardiol., 34,* 506, 1974.

9. Sinno, M. Z. and Gunnar, R. M.: Hemodynamic consequences of cardiac dysrhythmias. *Med. Clin. North Amer., 60,* 69, 1976.

10. Braun, H. A., Cheney, F. W., Loehnen, C. P.: Introduction to respiratory physiology. Little, Brown and Company, Boston, 1980.

5

Monitoring principles and equipment

To "monitor" is to watch. The nurse monitors many body processes, such as temperature, pulse, respiration, or blood pressure. In the CCU, the most important type of monitoring is continuous observation of the electrocardiogram.

Though many systems for monitoring the electrocardiogram are available, all have similar components and functions.

COMPONENTS OF ECG MONITORING

Electrode: Picks up small electrical currents produced by the heart.

Lead Wire: Carries the current from the electrodes to an amplifier.

Amplifier: Magnifies the small currents from the heart so they are large enough to be seen on a display apparatus, such as an oscilloscope, electrocardiograph, or rate meter.

45

Oscilloscope: A display apparatus in which an electron beam moves across the face of a tube, causing a glow where it strikes the tube. The ECG signal deflects the beam up and down, thus writing the ECG pattern.

Rate Meter: A device which counts the number of ventricular impulses and displays this rate on a meter. A sound or flash of light may be produced with each impulse.

Alarm: Integrated with the rate meter, the alarm can be set to give audible and visual warning at any preset low and high rate.

Electrocardiograph: An instrument which produces a written record of the ECG pattern. Some monitor systems automatically start the ECG when the alarm is triggered.

Most monitoring systems are designed so that the oscilloscope at the bedside can be attached to another oscilloscope, rate meter, and alarm at a remote site, such as a central nursing station. Such an arrangement allows monitoring of several beds from a single location. These remote oscilloscopes are often referred to as "slaves."

Electrodes

The electrical current generated by cardiac depolarization is distributed through the entire body. Thus, current generated in the heart can be picked up from any place in the body.

If electrodes on the body surface are to function well, the electrical resistance of the dry outer layers of skin must be reduced.

Skin resistance may be reduced by:

1. **Needle electrodes** penetrating the skin. Such electrodes are generally limited to emergency use.
2. **Electrode paste** on skin electrodes. The skin is initially scrubbed with alcohol to remove dry skin layers and skin oils. The electrode paste should be rubbed into the skin vigorously to further reduce skin resistance.

CORONARY CARE SYSTEM
Schematic Diagram

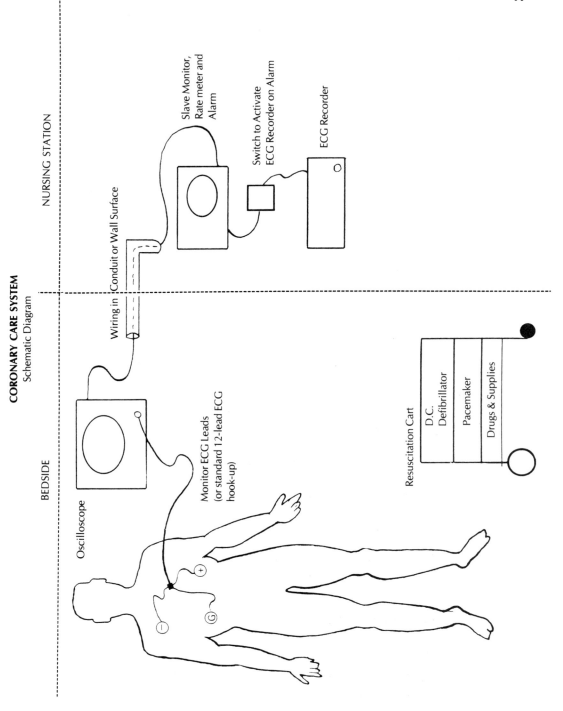

NURSING STATION

Slave Monitor, Rate meter and Alarm

Switch to Activate ECG Recorder on Alarm

ECG Recorder

Wiring in Conduit or Wall Surface

BEDSIDE

Oscilloscope

Monitor ECG Leads (or standard 12-lead ECG hook-up)

Resuscitation Cart

D.C. Defibrillator

Pacemaker

Drugs & Supplies

Electrode Placement

To obtain a routine, diagnostic 12-lead ECG, electrodes are placed on the extremities. Extremity electrodes are not satisfactory for constant monitoring.

1. The arms and legs become tangled in the cables.
2. It is difficult to work with the patient when wires are attached to the arms and legs.
3. The large muscle masses in the arms and legs produce considerable artifact.

Therefore, for monitoring, electrodes are placed on the chest, using a light-weight cable, usually with three electrodes. The electrodes usually are labeled:

Positive (or "left")
Negative (or "right")
Ground

Electrode Position

The following factors should be considered in selecting electrode position:

1. Electrodes must not interfere with the placement of paddles used for precordial shock.
2. Electrodes should be away from large muscle masses. Movement of skeletal muscles such as the pectorals will produce interference. This interference can be reduced by placing the electrodes over bony prominences such as the ribs.
3. Electrodes should be fairly close together to minimize tangling of wires.
4. The lead axis between the negative and the positive electrodes should be in the same general direction as the **Lead II axis,** i.e., from right to left and from head to foot.

The Lead II axis provides the best chance of recording a P wave and QRS complex of good amplitude.

Electrode Location:

Positive—Left lower chest, or just below the lowest rib, in the anterior axillary line.

Negative—Below the right clavicle, in the midclavicular line.

Ground—Right lower chest (although it could be placed anywhere).

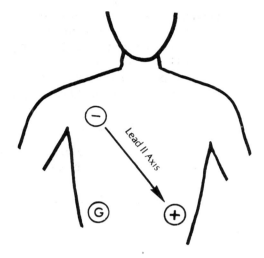

If the Lead II axis provides poor complexes:

1. Place the negative electrode in the right midaxillary line, in about the fourth intercostal space.
2. Place the positive electrode in the left midaxillary line, in about the fourth intercostal space.
3. Put the ground electrode any place on the right chest.
   or
4. Interchange the **negative** and **ground** electrode wires.

Modified Chest Lead (MCL-1 Lead)—Aberrant Conduction

The problem of differentiating VPC's from APC's with aberrant ventricular conduction has led some physicians to use a monitoring lead that helps to distinguish between these foci. Recall that a "different" QRS complex with prolonged duration may arise from:

1. **A Ventricular Focus**—Since the ectopic ventricular focus does not utilize the His-Purkinje system, but travels more slowly through ordinary myocardial muscle cells, the QRS complex will be wide, different, and prolonged in duration.

2. **A Supraventricular Focus with Aberrant Conduction**—A supraventricular focus usually utilizes the His-Purkinje system, producing a "narrow," normal-appearing QRS complex. However, if a portion of the His-Purkinje system is not functioning properly, part of the ventricular depolarization will be from myocardial muscle cell to cell, resulting in a "different" QRS complex with prolonged duration.

Usually aberrant conduction is due to absent or slowed conduction in the **right** bundle. Left bundle branch block also may produce aberrant conduction.

Right Bundle Branch Block—If delay is in the **right** bundle, the left ventricle is depolarized in a normal fashion. The right ventricle is depolarized late by the impulse traveling from myocardial muscle cell to cell. In general this late depolarization wave is directed anteriorly since the right ventricle lies anterior to the left.

Left Bundle Branch Block—The right ventricle is depolarized in a normal manner by the impulse traveling down the right bundle. The left ventricle is depolarized late by the impulse traveling from myocardial cell to cell. The general direction of this late depolarization is posterior since the left ventricle is posterior to the right ventricle.

A depolarization wave moving toward a positive electrode will produce a positive deflection in the ECG. A wave moving away from a positive electrode will produce a negative deflection.

The MCL-1 lead is a modified V1 monitoring lead.

Electrode Location:

Positive—Right anterior chest in approximately the V1 position, 4th interspace.

Negative—Left anterior chest, just below the clavicle in the midclavicular line.

Ground—Right anterior chest, just below the clavicle in the midclavicular line.

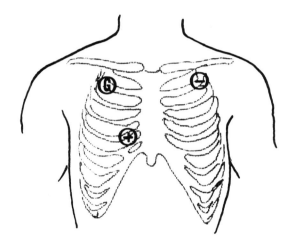

With the MCL-1 Monitoring Lead:

Aberrant ventricular conduction due to delay in the right bundle produces a positive deflection.

The occurrence of this right-bundle delay pattern is a hint that the anomalous QRS may be due to aberrant ventricular conduction.

The MCL-1 monitoring lead is useful in differentiating supraventricular ectopic beats and tachycardias with aberrant ventricular conduction from arrhythmias arising in the ventricles. This lead may not produce as large a P wave as the Lead II axis monitoring lead.

A five-electrode system with lead switch allows simple utilization of different leads:

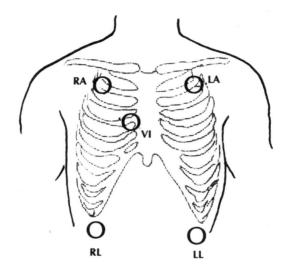

HINTS ON MONITORING

"Gain" Control

This control on the amplifier provides a means of increasing the magnification of the electrical signals. Increasing the gain will produce a taller tracing on the oscilloscope and may be helpful in identifying P waves. Too much gain may produce distortion which is difficult to interpret.

False Alarms

The rate meter measures the heart rate by counting the R waves of the ventricular complexes, and is integrated with the alarm.

Anything which alters the R wave may cause the alarm to sound:

1. **Low pattern**—Correct by relocating electrodes or increasing gain.
2. **Muscle interference**—Relocate electrode.
3. **Distortion with body movement**—Provide a tension loop in the electrode wire (page 54).
4. **Loose electrodes**—Reapply electrode.

Skin Care

The skin under the electrodes may become irritated after a period of monitoring. To avoid this, electrodes should be repositioned slightly every day or two. Frequent reapplication also helps to avoid loose electrodes and poor contact.

Troubleshooting

1. Produce a tension loop in the wire to prevent the transmission of tugging on the electrode. If the electrode moves on the skin, small currents are generated, causing artifact.
2. Excessive sweating: Use a stick deodorant to rub on the skin. Allow deodorant to dry completely and then place the electrodes as usual.
3. Shave the contact site.
4. Cleanse the site with alcohol.
5. Rub electrode paste thoroughly into the skin.
6. Use tincture of benzoin on the area where the adhesive device will be in contact with the skin.
7. Wash the electrodes thoroughly with soap and water to remove old electrode paste.
8. Needle electrodes may be used if there is difficulty from skin artifacts.

Tension Loop

A tension loop helps reduce artifact due to electrode motion.

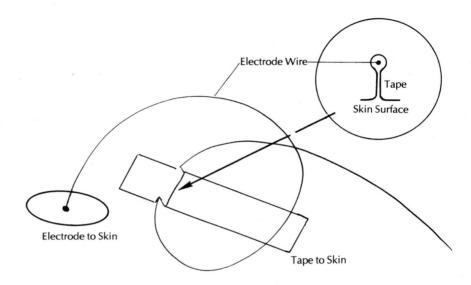

QUESTION SECTION—CHAPTER 5

1.	Electrical signals from the heart can be picked up by electrodes placed:	
	A. _____ On the arms.	
	B. _____ On the legs.	
	C. _____ On the chest.	
	D. _____ Anywhere on or in the body.	*D*
2.	In the CCU, the most important type of monitoring is continuous observation of the _____	*ECG.*
3.	Three ways to reduce skin resistance are:	
	A. _____ Shave the electrode site.	*A*
	B. _____ Clean the site with alcohol.	*B*
	C. _____ Scrub the site with soap.	
	D. _____ Rub the electrode paste into the skin.	*D*
4.	Muscle interference can be reduced by placing the electrodes over _____	*bony prominences.*
5.	Adhesive devices and a tension loop on the wire are used to avoid _____	*electrode movement.*

6. The image of the cardiac cycle on the oscilloscope can be made taller by:

A. _____ Changing the lead axis by repositioning the electrodes. *A*

B. _____ Using electrode paste.

C. _____ Increasing the gain on the amplifier. *C*

D. _____ Using needle electrodes.

---

7. The rate meter measures the rate of the:

_____ atria.

_____ ventricles. *ventricles.*

---

8. Check the items below that would help to avoid false alarms.

A. _____ Firmly applied electrodes.

B. _____ Application of electrodes over bony prominences.

C. _____ Tension loops in wires.

D. _____ Adequate height of R waves.

E. _____ Rubbing electrode paste into skin.

F. _____ Cleansing skin with alcohol.

G. _____ All of these. *G*

9. A wide "different" QRS complex may be produced by _____ and and _____ .	*ventricular focus supraventricular focus with aberrant ventricular conduction.*
10. In right bundle branch block, the _____ ventricle is depolarized last.	*right*
11. A depolarization wave moving toward a positive electrode produces a _____ deflection in the ECG.	*positive*
12. Aberrant ventricular conduction due to delay in the right bundle produces a _____ deflection in the MCL-1 lead.	*positive*
13. P waves usually are easiest to identify in: ____ MCL-1 lead. ____ Monitoring (II) lead.	*Monitoring (II) lead.*
14. Ectopy may be distinguished from aberration by using: ____ MCL-1 lead. ____ Monitoring (II) lead.	*MCL-1 lead.*

SUGGESTED READING—CHAPTER 5

1. Meltzer, L. E. and Dunning, A. J.: *Textbook of Coronary Care*. The Charles Press, Philadelphia, 1972.
2. Marriott, H. J. L. and Fogg, E.: Constant monitoring for cardiac dysrhythmias and blocks. *Mod. Concepts Cardiovasc. Dis., 39,* 103, 1970.

6

Arrhythmias complicating myocardial infarction

Detection and treatment of arrhythmias is a major duty of the CCU nurse.

The chief contribution of modern coronary care has been the prevention of arrhythmia deaths, previously the cause of nearly half the hospital deaths in myocardial infarction. Heart failure, shock, and other mechanical complications have not yet been greatly modified by new methods of management.

Catastrophic arrhythmias often can be prevented by prompt treatment of the minor arrhythmias which precede them.

CATASTROPHIC ARRHYTHMIAS	LESS SERIOUS ARRHYTHMIAS
Ventricular fibrillation	VPC's
Ventricular tachycardia	Atrial fibrillation
Ventricular standstill	Atrial flutter
Complete (third degree) A-V heart block	Supraventricular tachycardia
	APC's
	First degree A-V block
	Second degree A-V block

From a therapeutic standpoint, arrhythmias may be classified as:

Ectopic Rhythms—Arrhythmias which occur because of an abnormally excitable state of the myocardial tissue. Excitability may be enhanced by hypoxia, acidosis, hormones, drugs, and sympathetic stimulation.

Bradycardia, Block, and Escape Rhythms—Arrythmias produced by depression of normal pacemaker or conduction tissue. Foci with higher excitability than the depressed pacemaker or conduction tissue may then "escape" to produce an arrhythmia. Bradycardia and block may be produced by hypoxia, acidosis, drugs, and parasympathetic (vagal) stimulation.

ECTOPIC ARRHYTHMIAS	BRADYCARDIAS AND BLOCK
VPC's	Sinus bradycardia
Ventricular tachycardia	Junctional (nodal) rhythm
Ventricular fibrillation	First degree A-V block
APC's	Second degree A-V block
Atrial tachycardia	Third degree A-V block
Atrial flutter	Hemiblocks (fascicular blocks)
Atrial fibrillation	Ventricular standstill
Junctional (nodal) tachycardia	

ECTOPIC ARRHYTHMIAS

Ventricular Premature Contractions

VENTRICULAR PREMATURE CONTRACTIONS (VPC's)

Mechanism—Excitable focus in the ventricle.

Clinical Features—None, or sensation of palpitation or "skipping."

Significance—Increasing frequency may lead to ventricular tachycardia or fibrillation.

Treatment—Lidocaine, procainamide, quinidine, or Norpace®, especially if increasing in frequency, multiform, or in pairs. If ventricular rate is slow, speed rate with atropine or pacing.

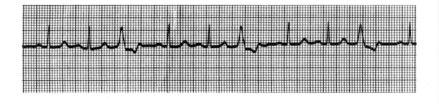

In acute myocardial infarction, all ventricular premature contractions (VPC's) are significant, but some are particularly dangerous because they warn of impending ventricular tachycardia or fibrillation.

CHARACTERISTICS OF PARTICULARLY DANGEROUS VPC's

1. Becoming more frequent as time passes.
2. Multifocal origin.
3. Occurring in pairs or triplets.
4. Constituting more than 10% of the QRS cycles or more than 5 per minute.

Ventricular Tachycardia

VENTRICULAR TACHYCARDIA

Mechanism—Excitable ventricular focus discharging repetitively.

Clinical Features—Apprehension, palpitation, signs of decreased cardiac output. Many episodes are brief, terminating spontaneously.

Significance—Dangerous, since it may terminate at any time in ventricular fibrillation or standstill.

Treatment—Try precordial thump precordial shock if tachycardia is prolonged or accompanied by circulatory collapse. Intravenous lidocaine, quinidine, or procainamide may terminate an attack and may prevent recurrence.

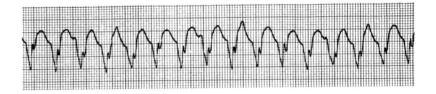

Ventricular tachycardia is an extremely dangerous arrhythmia. It reduces cardiac output and often is followed by ventricular fibrillation or standstill.

Brief runs of ventricular tachycardia may be treated with lidocaine. When sustained or associated with circulatory collapse, precordial shock (cardioversion) is the treatment of choice.

Ventricular Fibrillation

VENTRICULAR FIBRILLATION

Mechanism—Chaotic, uncoordinated, ineffective contractions of ventricular fibers.

Clinical Features—Syncope, apnea or gasping respirations, cyanosis, pulselessness, dilatation of pupils, convulsions.

Significance—Usually fatal if not treated within 3 to 4 minutes.

Treatment—Try precordial thump. Precordial shock is the first and often the only treatment needed in the CCU. If the initial shock is not successful, standard measures of CPR will be necessary.

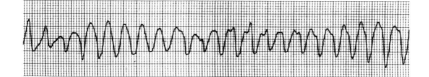

Individual myocardial fibers twitch, but there is no contraction and no cardiac output in this disorder. Without treatment, death soon results.

Secondary ventricular fibrillation describes this arrhythmia occurring secondary to profound shock or heart failure. Under these circumstances, ventricular fibrillation usually is fatal despite treatment; damage to the heart as a pump prevents successful treatment of the arrhythmia. Prevention of secondary ventricular fibrillation depends upon successful treatment of shock and heart failure; success is limited in both complications.

Primary ventricular fibrillation is less discouraging. This term is used to describe the arrhythmia occurring without antecedent shock or heart failure. In the CCU the mortality rate should be less than 2%, thanks to prompt recognition and treatment. In the general wards, recognition and treatment both are delayed; the mortality rate is at least 90%. Although defibrillation in the CCU is dramatically successful, it also is an admission of failure in prevention. Prevention of primary ventricular fibrillation is accomplished by treating the warning signs (see page 61) and other nonlethal arrhythmias which precede it.

Atrial Arrhythmias

Atrial arrhythmias often appear later in the course of acute myocardial infarction than ventricular arrhythmias, frequently in the second or third day. Though they superficially appear more benign than ventricular arrhythmias, atrial arrhythmias are associated with a high mortality rate probably because they are a sign of cardiac dilatation, low cardiac output, and congestive heart failure. They may also be a hint of some complicating factor, such as pulmonary embolism or drug intoxication. If they produce a rapid ventricular rate, atrial arrhythmias may increase cardiac work and decrease cardiac output.

Atrial Premature Contractions

ATRIAL PREMATURE CONTRACTIONS (APC's)

Mechanism—Excitable focus in atrium.

Clinical Features—Usually asymptomatic.

Significance—Atrial excitability may lead to more serious atrial arrhythmias.

Treatment—None if infrequent. Increasing frequency may require quinidine or procainamide. If signs of congestive heart failure, digitalis and diuretics may be indicated.

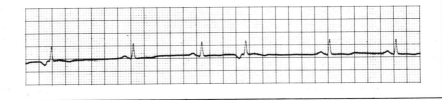

Atrial premature contractions are benign if infrequent. If common, new, or if increasing in frequency, they often warn of impending atrial tachycardia, flutter, or fibrillation.

Atrial Tachycardia

ATRIAL TACHYCARDIA

Mechanism—Excitable focus in the atrium, discharging repetitively.

Clinical Features—Sudden onset of rapid palpitation, feeling of fluttering in chest. May develop symptoms of shock, congestive failure, or angina. May terminate abruptly even without treatment.

Significance—An excessively rapid heart rate not only reduces cardiac output, but also increases cardiac oxygen requirements. Further myocardial damage, shock, or congestive failure may occur.

Treatment—Carotid sinus pressure may terminate atrial tachycardia. Digitalis, propranolol, quinidine, or procainamide also may be effective. Cardioversion is preferred if a fall in cardiac output produces angina, congestive failure, or shock. Consider digitalis toxicity, particularly if associated with block.

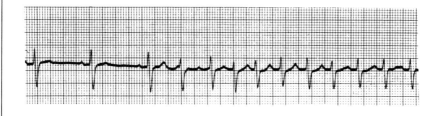

Atrial tachycardia can be serious since the rapid rate may reduce cardiac output and coronary blood flow (see page 24), causing further myocardial damage. Cardioversion is the treatment of choice if carotid sinus pressure is not promptly effective or if tachycardia produces chest pain, shock, or congestive failure. In less acute situations, drugs may be used to terminate this arrhythmia.

Atrial Flutter and Atrial Fibrillation

Atrial flutter and atrial fibrillation are important because cardiac output is reduced due to (1) the loss of atrial kick (see page 27) and (2) decreased ventricular filling. Both arrhythmias may be signs of congestive heart failure. They are often treated with digitalis or propranolol which slow the ventricular rate by reducing the number of atrial impulses transmitted by A-V junctional tissue. They may also be treated with cardioversion and are particularly responsive when of recent onset.

ATRIAL FLUTTER

Mechanism—Excitable atrial focus, discharging repetitively. Some degree of A-V block is usually present so that the ventricular rate is slower than the atrial rate.

Clinical Features—Patient may note palpitation with rapid ventricular rate. Asymptomatic if sufficient A-V block is present. Flutter waves may be seen in the neck veins.

Significance—Rapid ventricular rate may reduce cardiac output resulting in angina, myocardial damage, congestive failure, or shock.

Treatment—Cardioversion is preferred since atrial flutter often does not respond well to drugs. Digitalis or propranolol may be used to reduce A-V conduction. Quinidine may terminate atrial flutter.

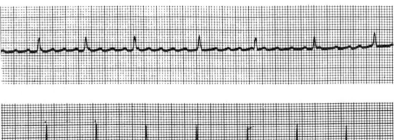

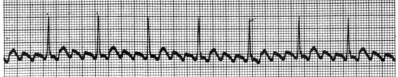

ATRIAL FIBRILLATION

Mechanism—Very rapidly discharging atrial foci. Only a portion of the atrial impulses is conducted through the A-V node to the ventricles. An irregular ventricular rhythm results.

Clinical Features—May be asymptomatic, or patient may note palpitation and irregularity. Radial pulse may be slower than apical rate (pulse deficit).

Significance—Cardiac output is reduced due to the irregular ventricular rhythm. There is more tendency for atrial thrombi and peripheral emboli. May be a sign of congestive heart failure.

Treatment—Digitalis or propranolol slow the ventricular rate by increasing A-V block. Quinidine or procainamide may convert atrial fibrillation to sinus rhythm. Cardioversion usually is successful in cases of recent onset.

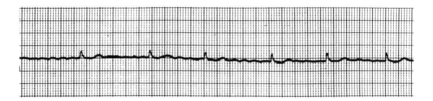

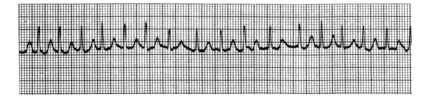

JUNCTIONAL (NODAL) TACHYCARDIA

Mechanism—Excitable focus in junctional tissue, which includes the A-V node and bundle of His. Special studies have shown that these arrhythmias arise from foci in the bundle of His rather than from the node itself.

Clinical Features—Sudden onset of palpitation, feeling of fluttering in chest. Similar to symptoms of atrial tachycardia, but since junctional tachycardia generally is slower, symptoms are less pronounced.

Significance—Often associated with digitalis intoxication. May produce increased myocardial work with reduced cardiac output and coronary blood flow.

Treatment—Withhold digitalis if being administered. If serum level is low, cautious administration of potassium may be helpful. Quinidine, procainamide, propranolol, or Dilantin may terminate. Cardioversion is contraindicated if arrhythmia is believed due to digitalis.

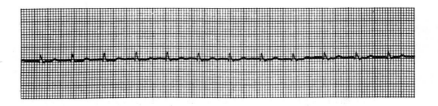

BRADYCARDIA AND BLOCK

SINUS BRADYCARDIA

Mechanism—Parasympathetic (vagal) stimulation of sinus nodal tissue frequently associated with inferior (diaphragmatic) myocardial infarction. Thrombosis involving the sinus node artery may produce ischemia of the sinus node.

Clinical Features—Often no symptoms. Slow ventricular rate may result in symptoms of low cardiac output such as angina, sweating, pallor, coolness, and mental obtundity.

Significance—Slow rate may seriously reduce cardiac output. "Escape" arrhythmias such as VPC's and ventricular tachycardia are enhanced.

Treatment—Atropine usually is effective. Pacing may be necessary if cardiac output is impaired or if escape arrhythmias occur.

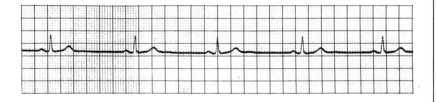

JUNCTIONAL (NODAL) RHYTHM

Mechanism—Depression of sinus node by vagal stimulation, ischemia, or drugs, with escape of focus in junctional tissues. Common as a manifestation of digitalis toxicity, where focus in junctional tissue may become more excitable (enhanced).

Clinical Features—Often no symptoms. Reduced cardiac output due to slow rate can produce symptoms of low output.

Significance—Slow ventricular rate may allow ventricular escape rhythms to develop.

Treatment—Atropine often is effective. Discontinue digitalis, quinidine, procainamide, lidocaine. Avoid use of these drugs for ectopic escape rhythms. Consider pacing if ventricular escape rhythms develop. Consider potassium for digitalis toxicity.

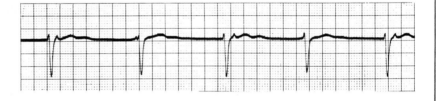

HEART BLOCK

Heart block is said to exist when the electrical wave of depolarization is delayed or stopped in its passage through the conducting system of the heart. Block may occur in the S-A node, atrial muscle, A-V node, junctional tissues, or bundle branches.

The A-V node, junctional tissue, and the bundle of His receive their blood supply from a branch of the right coronary artery. The right coronary artery also supplies the inferior (posterior) myocardium. Therefore, A-V block most commonly occurs in inferior myocardial infarction. A-V blocks arising from occlusion of the right coronary artery are ischemic in origin, worsen gradually, and are usually of short duration. If the block is second degree, it is usually of the Wenckebach type (Mobitz I), while if third degree, the escape rhythm usually arises in the junctional tissue with a relatively fast rate (50/min.) and narrow QRS configuration. The prognosis is good, and better with pacing.

A-V block may also occur with anterior or anteroseptal myocardial infarction. The right bundle, the anterior division (or "fascicle") of the left bundle, and a portion of the posterior branch of the left bundle receive their blood supply from branches arising from the anterior descending branch of the left coronary artery. If occlusion of the anterior descending artery produces extensive anteroseptal infarction, block may occur in one or more of these bundles. Thus block of the right bundle branch, the anterior or posterior fascicle of the left bundle branch (called "hemiblock"), or complete left bundle may occur.

Third degree, or "complete," block may occur if all three fascicles—the right bundle and the anterior and posterior fascicles of the left bundle—are interrupted ("trifascicular block"). This type of third degree A-V block, associated with extensive anteroseptal myocardial infarction, is accompanied by poor ventricular function, permanent block due to necrosis rather than ischemia, and poor prognosis, even with pacing. If the block is second degree, it is of the Mobitz II (not Wenckebach) type with a wide QRS configuration. If the block is third degree, the escape rhythm is from an idioventricular focus with a wide QRS configuration at a relatively slow rate (20 to 40/min.). Sudden arrest is common in trifascicular A-V block. *A-V block* may exist as the following.

First Degree A-V Block

Conduction through the A-V node is delayed, resulting in a PR interval of over 0.20 seconds. Each P wave is conducted.

FIRST DEGREE A-V BLOCK

Mechanism—Delay in conduction through the A-V node due to injury or drugs.

Clinical Features—None. Can be diagnosed by ECG only.

Significance—May be followed by an increase in the degree of A-V block.

Treatment—Usually observe. Consider atropine. Stop digitalis or quinidine if suspect.

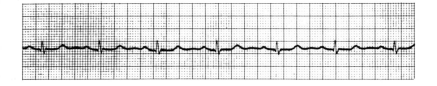

Second Degree A-V Block

Some of the atrial impulses are not conducted through the A-V node. The PR interval may be normal, prolonged, or variable.

SECOND DEGREE A-V BLOCK

Mechanism—Same as first degree A-V block, but some of the impulses are not transmitted through the A-V node.

Clinical Features—Often no symptoms. May be aware of slow ventricular rate.

Significance—May progress to third degree A-V block, ventricular arrhythmias, or standstill.

Treatment—Atropine. Prepare transvenous electrode for pacing. Discontinue digitalis, quinidine, propranolol, procainamide, lidocaine.

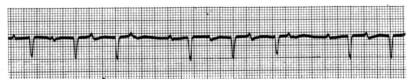

Second Degree A-V Block — Wenckebach (Mobitz I)

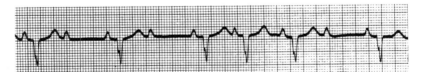

Second Degree A-V Block (Mobitz II)

Third Degree A-V Block

None of the impulses from the atria pass through the A-V node to reach the ventricles. This also is called *complete heart block.* The ventricles must begin their own inherent rhythm to continue circulation.

THIRD DEGREE A-V BLOCK

Mechanism—Same as first and second degree block. Injury to A-V node or fascicles. No atrial impulses reach the ventricles. A junctional or idioventricular pacemaker sustains ventricular contraction.

Clinical Features—May produce no symptoms. Adams-Stokes syncope may occur with slow rates or periods of brief asystole or ventricular fibrillation. Often produces shock, congestive heart failure.

Significance—Ventricular standstill or fibrillation may occur.

Treatment—Pacing.

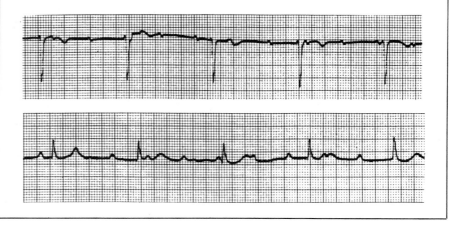

Characteristics of A-V Block in Acute Myocardial Infarction

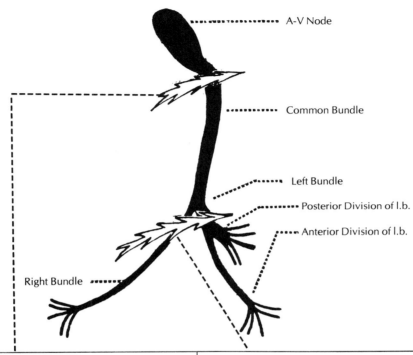

- A-V Node
- Common Bundle
- Left Bundle
- Posterior Division of l.b.
- Anterior Division of l.b.
- Right Bundle

HIGH BLOCKS (HERE)	LOW BLOCKS (HERE)
Due to A-V node injury.	Due to damage to both bundles or their divisions.
Prognosis good, better with pacing.	Prognosis poor, even with pacing.
Often transient (3–10 days), due to ischemia or edema.	Usually permanent, due to infarction (destruction) of conducting tissue.
More common with inferior infarction.	More common with extensive anteroseptal or multiple infarctions.
Ventricular function usually good.	Ventricular function usually poor.
ECG a. If second degree, usually Wenckebach type (Mobitz I) with narrow QRS. b. If third degree, escape rhythm usually is junctional, relatively fast (50/min.), narrow QRS.	ECG a. If second degree, Mobitz II (not Wenckebach) with wide QRS. b. If third degree, escape rhythm usually idioventricular, relatively slow (20–40/min.), wide QRS.

FEATURES WHICH ASSIST IN EVALUATION, PROGNOSIS AND NEED FOR PACING

Posterior Myocardial Infarction	Anterior Myocardial Infarction
Block common	Block rare
Block short-lived	Block lasts a long time or may be permanent
Escape QRS narrow	Escape QRS broad
Prognosis good (may be due to ischemia or small area of necrosis)	Prognosis poor (usually due to infarction of large area)

Second Degree A-V Block—Type I	Second Degree A-V Block—Type II
PR lengthens progressively until one P is not conducted, after which PR is shorter	Constant PR but some P waves are not conducted
QRS narrow	QRS in conducted cycles often somewhat broad
Gradually get worse or better	Suddenly get worse
Location of lesion junctional	Location of lesion in trifascicular system

Third Degree Block with QRS narrow	Third Degree Block with QRS Broad
Rate faster: 40–60/min.	Rate slower: 20–40/min.
Lesion less severe, may be ischemia or edema in junctional area	Lesion more severe, usually infarction, extensive area of septum
Outlook good if can be tided over brief period of bradycardia	Outlook poor, even with pacing, because of extensive muscle damage

VENTRICULAR STANDSTILL

Ventricular standstill may occur if the atria cease beating or atrial impulses are not conducted to the ventricles *and* a lower focus in the A-V node or ventricle does not arise. Standstill may result from drugs such as quinidine or excessive potassium. Failure of conduction of atrial impulses (third degree A-V block) may be due to myocardial damage or toxicity due to drugs.

During ventricular standstill, the electrocardiogram may demonstrate either no evidence of electrical activity or regularly occurring P waves without QRS complexes.

In many cases of ventricular standstill, no precipitating factor is apparent. In these "primary" situations, prompt treatment often is successful. When ventricular standstill is the result of prolonged shock or pulmonary edema or is "secondary" to other profound disturbances, it represents the terminal event; treatment is ineffective.

When a patient suffers sudden, unexpected ventricular standstill, the nurse's first step in treatment is a *vigorous blow to the precordium*. If this is ineffective in restoring the circulation within a few seconds, an artificial *pacemaker* should be activated if previously inserted. CPR should be instituted if no pacemaker is in place.

Increasing degrees of A-V block warn of the possibility of ventricular standstill. As a precautionary measure, the physician may insert a transvenous pacing catheter at the first sign of A-V conduction disorder. This permits prompt ventricular pacing, should ventricular standstill or complete (third degree) A-V block occur.

Treatment for ventricular standstill must begin immediately if it is to be effective.

VENTRICULAR STANDSTILL

Mechanism—Inadequate or absent electrical stimulus to produce ventricular contraction. Myocardial poisoning due to drugs.

Clinical Features—Same as ventricular fibrillation.

Significance—Fatal if not treated within a few minutes.

Treatment—Precordial blow, pacemaker, epinephrine, artificial respiration, and circulation.

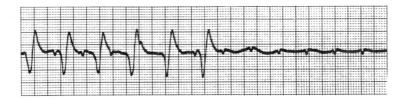

ILLUSTRATIVE CASES

1. A 54-year-old clerk. Inferior myocardial infarction one year previously. Admitted to CCU with one hour of severe retrosternal pain. ECG indicated acute anterior infarction.

   Monitor lead two hours after admission:

   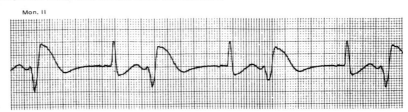

   Appropriate treatment would be:

   (1) _____ Procainamide, 0.5 gm. p.o.
   (2) _____ Lidocaine, 70 mg. I.V., followed by lidocaine drip, 2.0 mg./min.
   (3) _____ Atropine, 0.5–1.0 mg. I.V.

(2) is the correct choice. Lidocaine (Xylocaine®) is the drug of choice for treatment of ventricular premature contractions because of its rapid onset of action, low toxicity, and frequent effectiveness. Furthermore, when a drug is needed for prompt control of a significant arrhythmia, it should be given intravenously. Atropine might be used if the ventricular premature contractions were an "escape" phenomenon (see page 60). In this tracing, the sinus rate is 68 per minute. Note the P wave hidden in the ST segment of each VPC.

In this instance, the ventricular premature contractions were suppressed with a single bolus of lidocaine plus a lidocaine drip, which was gradually slowed over the next hour.

About two hours later, the following monitor pattern was noted:

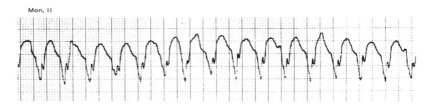

The patient noted palpitation, but the arrhythmia reverted to a sinus rhythm spontaneously after fifteen seconds.

What is the arrhythmia?

(1) ____ Sinus tachycardia with block
(2) ____ Atrial fibrillation
(3) ____ Ventricular tachycardia

(3) is the correct choice. Regular tachycardia with broad, different QRS complexes suggests ventricular tachycardia.

What would you do?

(1) ____ Observe the monitor carefully and give lidocaine, 70 mg. I.V. if further arrhythmias develop.
(2) ____ Give lidocaine 70 mg. I.V.
(3) ____ Start lidocaine drip, 2–4 mg./min.
(4) ____ Start quinidine 0.4 gm. q4h, or Pronestyl® 0.5 gm. q6h.

If you answered (1), review ventricular tachycardia again. Though it may subside spontaneously, ventricular tachycardia is likely to recur, to impair cardiac output, or to lead to further ventricular arrhythmias. If you simply observe the monitor, you may see this shortly:

Mon. II

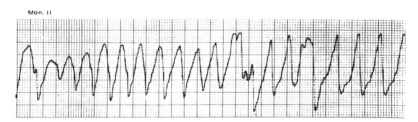

Answer (2) is correct. However if a lidocaine bolus is effective, it should be followed by an I.V. drip to maintain the level of lidocaine in the blood adequate to suppress the arrhythmia.

2. A 76-year-old male. Admitted to CCU after four hours of retrosternal pain, not relieved by nitroglycerin. Five-year history of typical angina. No previous ECG abnormality. ECG on admission showed acute anterior myocardial infarction. Nine hours after admission patient has recurrent pain, breathlessness, and palpitation. Blood pressure falls to 70/60.

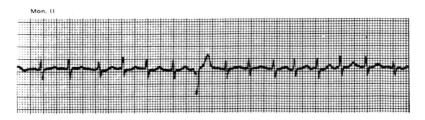

Mon. II

What is the arrhythmia?

(1) _____ Atrial fibrillation
(2) _____ Atrial tachycardia
(3) _____ Ventricular fibrillation

"Normal" appearing QRS complexes, irregular rhythm, and absence of P waves identify atrial fibrillation (1).

Here the nurse should notify the physician of the occurrence of atrial fibrillation and the symptoms. Pain, breathlessness, and hypotension all suggest a significant fall in the cardiac output. The physician may elect to give an intravenous digitalis preparation which will slow the ventricular rate by decreasing the number of atrial impulses which can traverse the A-V node. However, with symptoms suggesting significant fall in cardiac output, the physician may elect to use cardioversion and the nurse should be prepared to assist with this procedure without delay. (See Chapter 11.)

3. A 49-year-old mechanic admitted to CCU with ECG changes of acute inferior myocardial infarction. An intravenous catheter is introduced in an arm vein. Ten minutes later the alarm sounds and the monitor shows:

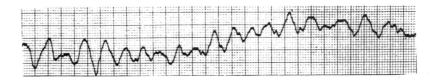

The nurse should:

(1) ___ Give lidocaine, 100 mg. I.V.
(2) ___ Give precordial shock at maximum voltage.
(3) ___ Start mouth-to-mouth breathing and external cardiac massage.

The treatment of ventricular fibrillation is prompt precordial shock (2). For this reason, every acute infarction patient should have a defibrillator at the bedside, turned on, ready for use. The sooner precordial shock is administered, the better the chance of success. Lidocaine would be administered after defribrillation to prevent recurrence. If initial shocks are not successful, CPR should be started.

4. A 62-year-old teacher hospitalized in CCU after development of retrosternal pain following extreme physical effort. ECG showed acute inferior myocardial infarction.

Mon. II

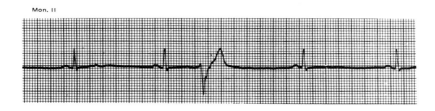

The nurse would give:

(1) ___ Morphine to relieve pain
(2) ___ Lidocaine, 70 mg. I.V.
(3) ___ Atropine, 1.0 mg. I.V.

Sinus bradycardia is common in early myocardial infarction. The slow rhythm may allow ectopic foci in the atria, the A-V node, or ventricles to "escape." Treatment should be directed to increasing the sinus rate with atropine (3). If ineffective, pacing may be needed. Trying to abolish "escape VPC's" with a depressant drug seldom is effective or safe.

If atropine were not effective, pacing may be used to increase the rate when frequent VPC's complicate sinus bradycardia.

5. A 50-year-old construction worker developed steady, burning discomfort deep to the midsternum which spread to the left shoulder, elbow, and forearm over the next two hours. Discomfort began to subside after four hours, and he drove seventy miles to the hospital. The ECG on admission showed an acute inferior myocardial infarction. PR on the first day was 0.18 second; second day, 0.24 second; and third day, 0.32 second.

    The following tracing was obtained.

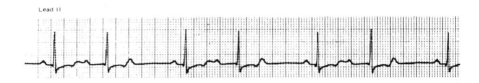

Which of the following might be done?

    (1) _____ Give atropine I.V.
    (2) _____ Give corticosteroid I.V.
    (3) _____ Stop quinidine.
    (4) _____ Insert transvenous pacing catheter.

Atropine was given intravenously without effect. Quinidine, being given for atrial premature contractions on the second day, was discontinued since this drug (and others—see Chapter 9) can prolong A-V conduction. In the meantime, the following change occurred:

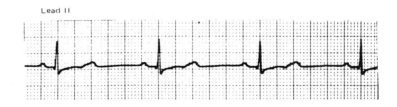

and a pacing catheter was introduced into the right ventricle with ECG guidance:

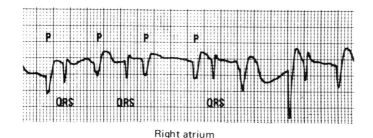

Right atrium

Intracardiac ECG with catheter tip in high right atrium. Note the large negative P wave.

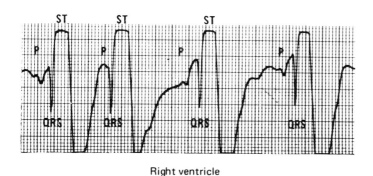

Right ventricle

Intracardiac ECG with tip of catheter touching right ventricular endocardium. Note the small P wave, large negative QRS, and marked ST elevation. The ST elevation occurs when the catheter tip touches the endocardium.

Pacing was instituted (see arrow).

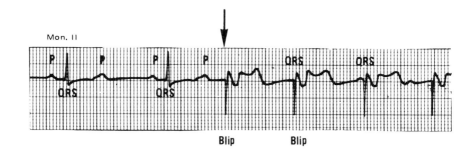

Monitoring lead from chest electrodes. The deep negative deflection is the pacing stimulus (blip). The QRS complex is wide and "different" since it arises from the pacing stimulus in the right ventricle.

QUESTIONS—CHAPTER 6

1. All infarction patients deserve and require skilled nursing care. The facilities of the CCU are designed particularly to prevent death from:

   A. Cerebral embolism.

   B. Ventricular standstill.   *B*

   C. Ventricular fibrillation.   *C*

   D. Pulmonary embolism.

   E. Shock.

   F. Congestive heart failure.

   G. Uremia.

2. Warning signs of impending circulatory arrest include:

   A. Increasing numbers of VPC's.   *A*

   B. Oliguria.

   C. Temperature above 100 degrees.

   D. Increasing PR interval.   *D*

   E. Multifocal VPC's.   *E*

   F. VPC's in pairs or triplets.   *F*

   G. VPC's superimposed on previous T wave.   *G*

   H. Bloody sputum.

   I. Third degree A-V block.   *I*

   J. More than 5 VPC's per minute.   *J*

3. List two factors which make it easier to prevent death from ventricular fibrillation in the CCU as contrasted with the general hospital floors:

   A. _____

   B. _____

A. *Prompt recognition due to monitoring by a skilled nurse.*

B. *Prompt treatment (defibrillation) by a trained nurse.*

4.

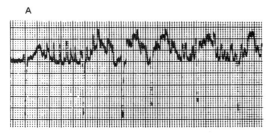

A. *Marked artifact, irregular ventricular rhythm of supraventricular origin.*

B. *Ventricular fibrillation.*

What are the chief features of the ECG strips shown above?

5. List the arrhythmias which are likely to progress to ventricular fibrillation:

A. _____   *Multifocal VPC's.*

B. _____   *VPC on T.*

C. _____   *Increasing VPC's.*

D. _____   *VPC's occurring more frequently than 5/min.*

E. _____

F. _____   *Runs of VPC's (brief runs of ventricular tachycardia).*

G. _____   *Ventricular tachycardia.*

Complete heart block (third degree).

---

6. Hypoxia, hyperpotassemia, excessive drugs, or increasing A-V block may result in _____ .   *ventricular standstill.*

---

7. During ventricular standstill, the electrocardiogram may show:

A. ____ Regularly-occurring P waves with slow or absent QRS complexes.   *A*

B. ____ Runs of VPC's.

C. ____ No electrical activity.   *C*

D. ____ Totally chaotic, irregular waves.

8. The first step in the treatment of ventricular standstill is _____ _____ _____ .

a vigorous blow to the precordium.

If this does not restore circulation within a few seconds, the next step is:

A. ____ Precordial shock.

B. ____ Activate the pacemaker.

B

---

9. Which of the following arrhythmias should be reported by the nurse?

A. ____ Multifocal VPC's.

A

B. ____ Wenckebach phenomena.

B

C. ____ Rare APC with aberration.

D. ____ Increasing A-V block.

D

E. ____ PR 0.26 sec.

E

---

10. What is the first action when ventricular standstill develops?

_____

Thump precordium

---

11. The above step has not been effective. The next action will be

_____

_____

activate the pacemaker, if inserted.

12. There is no response to the pacemaker. The nurse should now:

   A. _____ Give intracardiac epinephrine.

   B. _____ Begin ventilation and chest compression.   *B*

   C. _____ Give atropine I.V.

---

13. Atrial premature contractions usually are asymptomatic but should be treated if increasing in frequency because they:

   A. _____ Cause a decrease in cardiac output.

   B. _____ May lead to more serious atrial arrhythmias.   *B*

   C. _____ Can be confused with VPC's when aberrant conduction is present.

---

14. Atrial tachycardia may cause a decrease in cardiac output, producing angina, shock, or congestive heart failure. If carotid sinus pressure fails, the quickest way to terminate this arrhythmia is _____ _____ .

   cardioversion (precordial shock).

---

15. The ventricular rate in atrial flutter may be normal if _____ _____

   sufficient A-V block is present.

16. Atrial flutter often is treated with cardioversion. However, if a drug is used, the drug of choice for initial therapy is:

    A. Isoproterenol.

    B. Lidocaine.

    C. Digitalis.   *C*

    D. Quinidine.

---

17. Atrial fibrillation with a rapid ventricular rate may cause a low cardiac output because _____ _____ _____ .

    reduced diastolic period results in poor ventricular filling.

---

18. No response is noted in a patient with ventricular tachycardia when treated with lidocaine. The nurse would then _____ .

    prepare for precordial shock.

---

19. Ventricular tachycardia is dangerous because:

    A. ____ The rapid heart rate causes a fall in cardiac output.

    B. ____ Ventricular fibrillation or standstill commonly follows this arrhythmia.

    B

SUGGESTED READING—CHAPTER 6

1. Braun, H. A. and Diettert, G. A.: *ECG Arrhythmia Interpretation: A Programmed Text for Health Personnel.* Reston Publishing Co., Reston, Virginia, 1979.

2. Schamroth, L.: How to approach an arrhythmia. *Circulation, 47,* 420, 1973.

3. Marriot, H. J. L.: *Practical Electrocardiography,* Fifth Edition. Williams and Wilkins Co., Baltimore, 1972.

4. Uhley, H. N. The concept of trifascicular intraventricular conduction: Historical aspects and influence on contemporary cardiology. *Amer. J. Cardiol., 43,* 643, 1979.

5. Engel, T. R., Meister, S. G. and Frankl, W. S.: The "R-on-T" phenomenon. An update and critical review. *Ann. Intern. Med., 88,* 221, 1978.

6. Mullins, C. B. and Atkins, J. M.: Prognoses and management of ventricular conduction blocks in acute myocardial infarction. *Mod. Concepts Cardiovasc. Dis., 45,* 129, 1976.

7

Preservation of myocardium

Myocardial infarction results in necrosis of some myocardial cells because of loss of oxygen supply. These necrotic cells are surrounded by ischemic cells whose function is impaired and which could become necrotic if further oxygen demand develops.

One goal of the Coronary Care Unit is preservation of viable but ischemic myocardium by reducing myocardial oxygen consumption.

Myocardial oxygen consumption is related to:

1. Heart rate.
2. Myocardial contractility.
3. Ventricular wall tension.

HEART RATE

Sympathetic stimulation and catecholamines such as epinephrine and norepinephrine produce tachycardia. Anxiety, fever, and exertion produce tachycardia through these mechanisms. Myocardial infarction may result in tachycardia with abnormal rhythms. Treatment of tachycardia is directed toward the causative factors. Since oxygen supply is determined principally by blood flow, the reduced coronary blood flow associated with tachycardia and bradycardia may result in a disturbed balance between supply and demand.

An ischemic but viable myocardium may be preserved by control of tachycardia and bradycardia.

MYOCARDIAL CONTRACTILITY

Myocardial contractility may be thought of as the strength of the myocardial squeeze. Like tachycardia, sympathetic stimulation and increase in catecholamines increase myocardial contractility. Some drugs, such as isoproterenol, glucagon, and digitalis in the compensated heart, increase myocardial contractility and myocardial oxygen consumption. Beta-adrenergic blocking agents such as propanolol (Inderal) may be useful in decreasing myocardial contractility but must be used with caution as they can induce cardiac decompensation. At the present time, therapy is principally directed toward avoiding drugs which increase myocardial contractility.

VENTRICULAR WALL TENSION

Ventricular wall tension or stress refers to the pull on the myocardial muscle fibers and is related to both *left ventricular pressure* and *left ventricular volume*. Left ventricular pressure during systole, called "afterload," is related to the pressure the ventricle must pump against, or systolic blood pressure. Since increased afterload or hypertension results in increased myocardial oxygen consumption, it should be treated promptly.

Vasodilators, such as sodium nitroprusside, nitroglycerine, and isosorbide dinitrate, are being used increasingly since they reduce systolic pressure and left ventricular size and, therefore, ventricular wall tension.

Left ventricular pressure during diastole and left ventricular volume at end diastole are often referred to as "preload," and if increased, result in increased ventricular wall tension and increased myocardial oxygen consumption. Left ventricular end diastolic volume may be monitored by measuring the pulmonary capillary wedge pressure with a flow-directed catheter. Abnormally elevated pulmonary capillary wedge pressures are usually treated with diuretics, resulting in reduced left ventricular end diastolic filling pressure, left ventricular volume, and myocardial oxygen consumption.

Intra-aortic balloon pumping and external counterpulsation are mechanical devices which reduce both preload and afterload, and increase coronary blood flow. Their use, however, is limited to occasional patients with cardiogenic shock or congestive heart failure unresponsive to other therapy (see Chapter 8).

Administration of supplemental oxygen increases diffusion of oxygen into ischemic areas in animal experiments, reducing infarct size. Though this has not been confirmed in humans, it seems reasonable to administer supplemental oxygen to patients with acute infarctions.

Still unproven maneuvers to reduce infarct size include administration of glucose, insulin, and potassium solutions, presumably improving myocardial energy supply, and administration of corticosteroids, which may reduce cellular damage due to release of local toxins. Their routine use is not recommended at this time.

SUGGESTED READING—CHAPTER 7

1. Helfant, R. H., Banka, V. S. and Bodenheimer, M. M.: Perplexities and complexities concerning the myocardial infarction border zone and its salvage. *Amer. J. Cardiol., 41,* 345, 1978.

2. Jennings, R. B. and Reimer, K. A.: Salvage of ischemic myocardium. *Mod. Concepts Cardiovasc. Dis., 43,* 125, 1974.

3. Maroko, P. R., Radvany, P., Braunwald, E., and Hale, S. L.: Reduction in infarct size by oxygen inhalation following acute coronary occlusion. *Circulation, 52,* 360, 1975.

4. Braunwald, E. and Maroko, P. R.: Reduction of infarct size—an idea whose time (for testing) has come. *Circulation, 50,* 206, 1974.

5. Hearse, D. J., Opie, L. H., Katzeff, I. E., *et al.:* Characterization of the "border zone" in acute regional ischemia in the dog. *Amer. J. Cardiol., 40,* 716, 1977.

6. Hoffman, J. I. E. and Buckberg, G. D.: The myocardial supply: demand ratio—a critical review. *Amer. J. Cardiol., 41,* 327, 1978.

7. Sonnenblick, E. H. and Skelton, C. L.: Oxygen consumption of the heart: Physiological principles and clinical implications. *Mod. Concepts Cardiovasc. Dis., 40,* 9, 1971.

8. Epstein, S. E., Kent, K. M., Golstein, R. E., Boyer, J. S. and Redwood, D. R.: Reduction of ischemic injury by nitroglycerine during acute myocardial infarction. *N. Eng. J. Med., 292,* 29, 1975.

9. Hutchins, G. M. and Bulkley, B. H.: Infarct expansion versus extension: Two different complications of acute myocardial infarction. *Amer. J. Cardiol., 41,* 1127, 1978.

8

Mechanical complications of myocardial infarction

The complications of myocardial infarction may be classified as *electrical* or *mechanical*. Electrical complications, the arrhythmias, are more responsive to treatment than mechanical complications considered in this chapter. Development of the CCU has done little to improve the prognosis in patients with mechanical complications of acute myocardial infarction.

Mechanical complications include:

1. EMBOLISM
2. VENTRICULAR RUPTURE
3. MITRAL VALVE INSUFFICIENCY
4. CONGESTIVE HEART FAILURE
5. SHOCK

EMBOLISM

Pulmonary Embolism

Pulmonary embolism occurs more commonly than suspected. Autopsy studies show pulmonary emboli in about 25% of myocardial infarction fatalities, but they are the direct cause of death in only 10%. The blood clot responsible for pulmonary embolism usually has formed in the deep veins of the legs, especially when the rate of blood flow is slowed because of poor cardiac action, inactivity of the legs, dependency, and previous phlebitis. A portion of the clot travels quickly from the legs to the heart and then is stopped when it reaches the small branches of a pulmonary artery. *Pulmonary infarction* is the result of interruption of blood flow to the lungs caused by an embolism. Although the patient may have no symptoms or only minor symptoms from his first, small pulmonary embolism, later or larger emboli are likely to cause congestive failure, sudden breathlessness, pleuritic chest pain (chest pain accentuated by respiration), hemoptysis, and shock.

The *prevention of pulmonary embolism* is accomplished by anticoagulant therapy. The chief benefit of anticoagulant therapy is prevention of clots in the leg veins *(phlebothrombosis),* rather than an effect on the coronary artery thrombosis. Additional preventive measures include elastic stockings, leg exercise, frequent change of position, avoidance of obstruction in the popliteal fossae from use of the Gatch bed, and preventing long periods of dependency of the legs.

PULMONARY EMBOLISM

1. Common, often overlooked.
2. Thrombi released from leg veins, right ventricle, or pelvic veins.
3. Symptoms range from none to dyspnea, pleuritic pain, heart failure, shock, and hemoptysis.
4. Prevention:
   a. Anticoagulants
   b. Elastic stockings
   c. Leg exercises
   d. Change in position
   e. Avoid popliteal obstruction

NURSING RESPONSIBILITIES IN
PULMONARY EMBOLISM

Prevention: Proper application of elastic stockings. Leg exercises. Frequent changes in body position. Avoidance of obstruction in the popliteal fossae by the Gatch bed or pillows. Avoidance of long periods of dependent position of legs.

Arterial Embolism

Myocardial infarction involves the inner lining of the heart (endocardium) as well as the heart muscle itself. The raw, necrotic endocardium is a common site of clot formation *(mural thrombus)*. If the interventricular septum is involved, a mural thrombus may form in the right ventricle, breaking off to lodge in the lungs. Mural thrombi are more common in the left ventricle, the site of most myocardial infarctions. A clot which breaks off from a mural thrombus in the left ventricle will pass out the aorta, lodging in one of its branches to the brain, kidney, or lower extremities and causing an *arterial embolism*. Prevention of mural thrombi is attempted through the use of anticoagulants.

EMBOLISM FROM MURAL THROMBUS

1. Uncommon.
2. Thrombus formed on area of infarction, released into systemic circulation.
3. Sudden signs of interruption of arterial circulation (such as stroke, abdominal pain, pallor, pain, and absence of pulse in extremity).
4. Prevention: Anticoagulants.

NURSING RESPONSIBILITIES IN EMBOLISM
FROM MURAL THROMBUS

Prompt recognition of signs of arterial obstruction:

1. Pain, pallor, pulselessness in an extremity.
2. Stroke: Hemiparesis, change in mental status.

VENTRICULAR RUPTURE

Ventricular rupture ordinarily is untreatable and fortunately is rare. It usually occurs with an extensive infarction in which there is a large area of necrosis extending completely through the ventricular wall. The time of occurrence of rupture most commonly is from the fifth to the tenth day when the necrotic area is weakest. When rupture occurs, blood fills the pericardial sac, producing *tamponade* (compression) of the heart. This prevents cardiac filling; death quickly ensues.

There are *two points of practical significance* regarding ventricular rupture. *First is prevention. Anticoagulant therapy* may contribute to rupture and should be avoided when patients with transmural infarction develop a friction rub or symptoms of *pericardial irritation. A friction rub* is a loud, grating sound heard over the heart during systole and diastole. When the pericardium is irritated by the necrosis beneath it, often there is recurrence of chest pain. However, the pain of pericardial irritation differs from the original pain of the infarction. The discomfort is likely to be accentuated by breathing or by rolling onto one side or the other. Often it is associated with tenderness of the precordium. Rupture also is more common in patients who exercise unwisely during the early days following infarction.

The *second practical point* is to distinguish rupture from treatable causes of circulatory arrest, such as ventricular standstill or fibrillation. The patient dying suddenly with rupture is likely to have a satisfactory ECG rhythm without palpable pulse, at least during the early minutes. Sudden distention of the neck veins also may be a clue to the diagnosis of rupture.

VENTRICULAR RUPTURE

1. Rare, usually untreatable.
2. Perforation of ventricle with release of blood into pericardial sac.
3. Sudden death, not preceded by arrhythmia. Distinguish from treatable causes of sudden death.
4. Prevention:
   a. Avoid premature activity.
   b. Stop anticoagulants if friction rub develops.

NURSING RESPONSIBILITIES IN VENTRICULAR RUPTURE

1. *Prevention.* Recognition of pericardial pain, often pleuritic in nature, may be a clue. Avoid unwise exercise of patient with transmural infarction.
2. *Distinguish from treatable causes of sudden death.* Cardiac arrest due to ventricular fibrillation or standstill should be recognized and treated promptly. Ventricular rupture is not often associated with an arrhythmia. Sudden extreme distention of the neck veins may be a clue in ventricular rupture.

Ventricular rupture also may occur as a rupture of the ventricular septum, usually in association with an extensive anteroseptal myocardial infarction. Septal rupture may be suspected when there is sudden development of a loud precordial systolic murmur and signs of congestive heart failure.

The sudden development of a defect in the septum, with shunting of blood from the left ventricle to the right usually results in a large increase in left ventricular work and left ventricular failure, usually unresponsive to medical therapy. A flow-directed balloon catheter in the pulmonary artery is mandatory for evaluation of medical therapy in these patients. Surgical closure of the defect, though associated with a high mortality, is the only therapeutic hope.

MITRAL VALVE INSUFFICIENCY

The mitral valve is connected to the papillary muscles by the chordae tendineae. Contraction of the papillary muscles with tightening of the chordae permits precise closure of the mitral valve during systole. Infarction may involve the chordae or papillary muscles, in which case mitral closure may be imperfect. During systole, blood in the left ventricle regurgitates into the left atrium, resulting in a systolic murmur, increased left ventricular work, and reduced left ventricular efficiency. If the regurgitant volume is large, congestive heart failure resistant to medical therapy may result.

Necrosis of the papillary muscle due to infarction may result in separation of the attachment of the chordae tendineae from the papillary muscle. Severe mitral insufficiency is associated with a loud systolic murmur and profound congestive heart failure. Again, measurements of pulmonary artery and pulmonary capillary wedge pressures are necessary for guiding medical therapy.

Surgical correction of mitral valve insufficiency due to either papillary muscle dysfunction or chordae tendineae separation may be of value if the patient responds to medical therapy sufficiently to tolerate the surgical procedure.

CONGESTIVE HEART FAILURE

Congestive heart failure is present when one or both ventricles are unable to empty adequately during systole; the volume of blood and pressure in the ventricles are elevated during diastole. When the left ventricle fails, blood backs up into the lungs, distending the pulmonary veins and capillaries. Plasma may leak into the air sacs (alveoli), producing pulmonary edema. If left ventricular failure occurs acutely, as often happens in myocardial infarction, sudden severe dyspnea, cyanosis, gurgling breathing, cough, frothy pink sputum, and shock may develop. Tachycardia, S-3 gallop, cardiac enlargement, and elevated pulmonary wedge pressure are other common findings.

The occurrence of acute left ventricular failure with pulmonary edema in acute myocardial infarction usually indicates extensive myocardial damage and has a poor prognosis. Measurement of pulmonary wedge pressures is helpful in management after initial emergency therapy.

Treatment of acute pulmonary edema is aimed at reducing the amount of blood returning to the heart.

1. *Rotating tourniquets, phlebotomy,* and the *seated position* reduce the amount of blood returning to the heart. Vasodilators such as nitroglycerin, nitrates, and nitroprusside may be indicated.
2. *Diuretics* result in excretion of retained sodium and water.
3. *Oxygen* and *digitalis* improve the heart pumping ability.
4. *Sedation,* with relief of apprehension, reduces cardiac work.

Another common form of congestive heart failure develops more slowly. Decreased cardiac output results in decreased circulation to the kidneys. The kidneys respond by retaining sodium and water, thereby increasing the blood volume.

The development of chronic congestive heart failure in a patient with acute myocardial infarction usually occurs after several days. It also indicates severe left ventricular dysfunction and has a poor prognosis.

Chronic congestive heart failure results in dyspnea, and signs of fluid retention, which may include weight gain, increased venous pressure, and fluid collection in the lungs, liver, abdomen, and legs.

Treatment again includes digitalis to improve cardiac pumping. Sodium and water retention are combated with sodium restriction and diuretic drugs which stimulate the kidneys to excrete the excessive sodium and water. Vasodilators pool blood peripherally, reduce venous return, and lower systemic blood pressure.

Though digitalis is an extremely useful drug, an excess may produce toxic symptoms. These include anorexia, nausea and vomiting, and arrhythmias. The drug should be stopped if digitalis intoxication is suspected.

Diuretics, if used too vigorously, may result in hypovolemia. Hypokalemia is commonly produced if adequate replacement is not provided. Hypokalemia in the presence of digitalis, hypoxia, acidosis, or alkalosis may result in serious ventricular arrhythmias.

Vasodilator therapy is frequently monitored with measurement of both systemic and pulmonary capillary wedge pressures to assure adequate left ventricular filling pressure and systemic blood pressure.

CONGESTIVE HEART FAILURE

1. Ventricle(s) fails to empty fully.
2. Dyspnea, peripheral edema.
3. Prevention:
   a. Avoid salt.
   b. Avoid activity.
4. Measure pulmonary artery and pulmonary capillary wedge pressures and pulmonary artery oxygen saturation as guides to therapeutic interventions.
5. Treat with rest, oxygen, diuretics, digitalis, and vasodilators such as nitroglycerin, nitrates, nitroprusside, hydralazine, and prazosin.

NURSING RESPONSIBILITIES IN CONGESTIVE HEART FAILURE

1. Accurate weight and measurement of intake and output.
2. Restrict sodium in diet. Well-meaning visitors often try to help the ill patient by bringing favorite foods.
3. Avoid excessive activity.
4. Rotating tourniquets, oxygen, seated position, and sedation in acute left ventricular failure.
5. Monitoring pulmonary capillary wedge pressure, pulmonary artery pressure, systemic blood pressure, and pulmonary artery oxygen saturation.

SHOCK

The heart with a recent infarction does not pump efficiently. A profound decrease in the cardiac output may occur. If tissue perfusion is inadequate, the situation is called *cardiogenic shock.* Congestive failure often precedes or accompanies shock.

Although hypotension is one of the cardinal signs of shock, the fundamental derangement is inadequate tissue perfusion. Thus, elevation of blood pressure may not cure cardiogenic shock. The basic need is to increase blood flow.

Other signs of shock result from vasoconstriction or from inadequate flow of blood to various organs.

Skin and Muscles: Pallor, coolness, cyanosis, sweating, fatigue.

Kidneys: Oliguria, sodium and fluid retention.

Brain: Lethargy, coma, agitation, confusion.

Heart: Hypotension, heart failure, arrhythmias, angina, further infarction.

Cardiogenic shock is due to poor pumping. However, pump failure is not the only cause of shock in myocardial infarction. *Hypovolemia* may be a contributing factor. The acute infarction patient may have a considerable fluid deficit due to sweating, vomiting, and low intake. Bleeding may complicate excessive anticoagulant effect. Proper assessment of fluid balance and replacement of losses will reverse hypovolemic shock. The determination of the pulmonary diastolic pressure, pulmonary capillary wedge pressure, and pulmonary artery oxygen saturation (see Chapter 4) are particularly helpful in the diagnosis and treatment of shock.

Tachycardia, bradycardia, and other arrhythmias likewise may precipitate cardiogenic shock.

CARDIOGENIC SHOCK

Cardiogenic shock has a poor prognosis with a fatality rate of about 80%. It usually represents a loss of 40% or more of functional myocardium. Certain measures may be of value in selected cases:

1. *General measures.* Oxygen may help the depressed myocardium and improve cardiac output, especially if pulmonary complications have produced hypoxia. Pain medication should be used cautiously as its excretion may be slowed and respiratory depression and peripheral vasodilation may be produced.

2. *Measurement of left ventricular filling pressure and cardiac output.* Pulmonary capillary wedge pressure measurement with a flow-directed balloon catheter is mandatory. A low wedge pressure suggests hypovolemia as a cause of hypotension, and fluid replacement, as colloid or cystalloid, may correct shock. Maintenance of the wedge pressure at 15–20 mm. Hg. may improve cardiac output. If high, wedge pressure may respond to phlebotomy, diuretics, or vasodilators. Pulmonary artery oxygen saturation reflects cardiac output, and relative changes may help in evaluation of therapeutic maneuvers.

3. *Vasopressors.* Dopamine (Intropin®) is usually the initial vasopressor used. In small to moderate doses, it improves myocardial contraction and perfusion of the kidneys and gut. Systemic vascular resistance may be decreased or unchanged.

If inadequate response is obtained with dopamine, a trial of *levarterenol* (Levophed®) or *metaraminol* (Aramine®) may be indicated. These drugs not only increase cardiac output but also systemic peripheral resistance and may, therefore, detrimentally increase myocardial work.

4. *Vasodilators.* If systemic peripheral resistance is elevated, vasodilators may improve cardiac output by decreasing myocardial work. Vasodilators are generally used with vasopressors, balancing dosage by measurements of wedge pressure, pulmonary artery oxygen saturation, and systemic blood pressure, and calculation of systemic vascular resistance:

$$\frac{\text{(mean arterial pressure)}}{\text{(cardiac output estimated from pulmonary artery oxygen saturation)}}.$$

Vasodilators such as *sodium nitroprusside* (Nipride®), nitroglycerin, long acting nitrates, hydralazine (Apresoline®), or *prazosin* (Minipress®) are most useful when left ventricular filling pressure is high. Though cardiac output may be improved, peripheral vasodilation may aggravate hypotension and decrease tissue perfusion.

5. *Diuretics.* Intravenous furosemide (Lasix®) is often used with elevated left ventricular filling pressures.

6. *Digitalis.* There is no clear-cut evidence that digitalis is helpful in cardiogenic shock though it is of value in left ventricular failure associated with left ventricular dilatation. Cardiogenic shock represents a form of profound left ventricular failure.

7. *Arrhythmias.* Correction of bradycardia, tachycardia, or other arrhythmias may improve cardiac output.

8. *Mechanical-assist devices.* Intra-aortic balloon pumping (IABP) is the most commonly used mechanical support technique. A balloon, positioned in the descending aorta, is timed by the electrocardiogram to inflate at the onset of diastole, and deflate just before systole, reducing afterload and myocardial work, and improving coronary and cerebral blood flow. The use of IABP for cardiogenic shock has been disappointing though most patients improve clinically. Its use should be limited to those patients who may have a surgically treatable lesion such as post-infarction ventricular septal defect, mitral insufficiency due to papillary muscle rupture, or the rare patient with shock due to profound left ventricular ischemia without infarction. IABP allows temporary stabilization so that left ventriculography and coronary arteriography can be performed.

NURSING RESPONSIBILITIES IN SHOCK

1. *Accurate determination of blood pressure.* Faulty technique or defective equipment may lead to a mistaken diagnosis. The artery where blood pressure is measured should be at the level of the heart. Cuff pressure should not be lowered too rapidly or too slowly. In some patients, the sounds disappear as the pressure is lowered and reappear above the diastolic pressure; this is known as "auscultatory gap." Blood pressure determinations using the manometer are frequently erroneous during shock. Direct measurement with an intraluminal needle and an electronic gauge (transducer) often is preferred. Check the systolic pressure by palpation of the artery. Look for other signs of shock besides hypotension.

2. *Accurate measurement of pulmonary capillary wedge pressure or pulmonary diastolic pressure.*

3. *Accurate measurement of fluid intake and urine output.* Where available, a bed scale for weighing is helpful. A change in weight of 1 kilogram is equal to a change in fluid balance of 1000 cc. A urinometer helps to measure hourly urine volume.

4. *Administer oxygen.*

5. *Control rate of administration of vasopressors* to maintain adequate blood pressure. Vasopressors may cause side effects such as arrhythmias, extracellular fluid depletion with further hypotension, or excessive vasopressor response. Problems may be further complicated with the addition of vasodilators.

6. *Recognize early signs and symptoms* of decreased tissue perfusion (see page 102). An early, aggressive attack on treatable factors such as arrhythmias, hypoxemia, hypovolemia, and congestive heart failure may prevent the easily recognized and nearly hopeless full-blown picture of cardiogenic shock.

QUESTIONS—CHAPTER 8

1. A mild degree of congestive heart failure is common following myocardial infarction. What dietary order is designed to minimize its severity?
   _____

   Sodium restriction

2. The causes of fluid retention following myocardial infarction include:

   A. Renal emboli.

   B. Decreased renal blood flow.   *B*

   C. Liquid diet.

   D. Excessive drinking water.

   E. I.V. drip.

   F. Reduced cardiac output.   *F*

3. Leg exercises, frequent changes of body position, compression stockings, and anticoagulants help prevent leg vein
   _____ .

   thrombosis

4. A clot breaks away from a calf vein. From the choices below list in proper sequence the structures through which it will pass.

Cerebral arteries

Pulmonary vein

Right atrium

Right ventricle

Femoral vein

Pulmonary artery

Aorta

Inferior vena cava

1. *Femoral vein*

2. *Inferior vena cava*

3. *Right atrium*

4. *Right ventricle*

5. *Pulmonary artery*

---

5. A clot originating in a leg vein and lodging in a branch of the pulmonary artery is called a _____ .

pulmonary embolism

---

6. Obstruction of a pulmonary artery by an embolus produces:

A. Atelectasis.

B. Pneumonia.

C. Pulmonary infarction.

D. Pulmonary edema.

C

7. List four measures which help prevent peripheral thrombophlebitis and secondary pulmonary emboli:

    A. _____   *Leg exercises*

    B. _____   *Elastic wraps or stockings*

    C. _____   *Frequent changes of*
                                    body position
    D. _____   *Anticoagulants*

8. A mural thrombus is released from the left ventricle, producing a stroke by cerebral embolism. From the choices below, list in order the vascular structures through which it will pass.

    Mitral valve   *1. Aortic valve.*

    Aortic valve   *2. Aorta.*

    Pulmonary vein   *3. Carotid artery.*

    Superior vena cava   *4. Cerebral artery.*

    Carotid artery

    Cerebral artery

    Pulmonary artery

    Aorta

9. The principal prophylactic measure for prevention of emboli from mural thrombi is_____ .   *anticoagulation.*

10. Shock in myocardial infarction is due to:

   A. Low blood volume.

   B. Bacterial infection.

   C. Inadequate cardiac function.   C

---

11. List some signs and symptoms of shock:

   A. _____   *Hypotension*

   B. _____   *Pale, cool, sweaty skin*

   C. _____   *Oliguria*

   D. _____   *Restlessness, mental confusion, coma*

---

12. Erroneously low blood pressure readings can be minimized by using:

   A. A mercury manometer.

   B. A snug cuff.

   C. Proper technique.   C

13. Indicate the action of the following therapeutic measures:

A. _____ Oxygen.

B. _____ Digitalis.

C. _____ Elevation of the foot of bed.

D. _____ Vasopressors.

1. Improves the return of blood to the heart.

2. May increase the force of cardiac contraction.

3. May produce arrhythmias.

4. Decreases the volume of the vascular bed.

A. 2

B. 2, 3

C. 1, 2

D. 1, 4

14.

What is the rhythm in this ECG which is commonly seen in shock?

_____

This is a reflex tachycardia because of poor cardiac output. What treatment might be of value?

_____

_____

_____

_____

Sinus tachycardia (bundle branch block is present)

Digitalis

Oxygen

Elevation of the foot of the bed

Vasopressors

15. Acute pulmonary edema is treated by utilizing two principles:

    A. Reduction of venous return.

    B. Improvement of cardiac pumping.

    Which principle is involved in the following therapeutic measures:

    ____ 1. Rotating tourniquets.   *A*

    ____ 2. Digitalis.   *B*

    ____ 3. Oxygen.   *B*

    ____ 4. Morphine.   *A*

    ____ 5. Sitting position.   *A*

16. Diuretics and sodium restriction prevent retention of:

    A. Calcium.

    B. Sodium.   *B*

    C. Glucose.

    D. Water.   *D*

17. Digitalis is helpful in the treatment of congestive heart failure because it:

    A. Causes loss of appetite.

    B. Improves cardiac pumping.   *B*

    C. Causes sodium excretion.

    D. Increases cardiac output.   *D*

    E. Slows the heart rate.   *E*

---

18. Excess digitalis may cause anorexia, nausea, vomiting, and ventricular premature contractions.

    Appropriate treatment would be _____ .   *stop the digitalis.*

19. Inadequate cardiac output may produce:

    A. Angina.

    B. Lethargy.

    C. Syncope.

    D. Hypotension.

    E. Confusion.

    F. Pallor.

    G. Sweating.

    H. Fluid retention.

    I. Apprehension.

    J. Decreased urine volume.

    K. Belligerence.

    L. Coma.

    M. Convulsion.

    N. Weakness.

    O. Easy fatigue.

    P. All of the above.

P

20. Of the signs included in Question 19, list those which are due to inadequate circulation to the:

   1. Heart   _____   *A, D*

   2. Brain   _____   *B, C, E, I, K, L, M*

   3. Kidney   _____   *H, J*

   4. Skin and muscles   _____   *F, G, N, O*

SUGGESTED READING—CHAPTER 8

1. Bates, R. J., Beutler, S., Resnekov, L. and Anagnostopoulous, C. E.: Cardiac rupture-challenge in diagnosis and management. *Amer. J. Cardiol., 40,* 429, 1977.

2. Kleiger, R., Shaw, R. and Avioli, L. V.: Postmyocardial complications requiring surgery. *Arch. Intern. Med., 137,* 1580, 1977.

3. Chalmers, T. C., Matla, R. J., Smith, H., Jr. and Kunzler, A. M.: Evidence favoring the use of anticoagulants in the hospital phase of acute myocardial infarction. *N. Eng. J. Med., 297,* 1091, 1977.

4. Luepker, R. V., Caralis, D. G., Voigt, G. C., Burns, R. L., Murphy, L. W. and Warbasse, J. R.: Detection of pulmonary edema in acute myocardial infarction. *Amer. J. Cardiol., 39,* 146, 1977.

5. Forrester, J. S., Diamond, G. S. and Swan, H. J. C.: Correlative classification of clinical and hemodynamic function after acute myocardial infarction. *Amer. J. Cardiol., 39,* 137, 1977.

6. Chatterjee, K. and Swan, H. J. C.: Vasodilator therapy in acute myocardial infarction. *Mod. Concepts Cardiovasc. Dis., 43,* 119, 1974.

7. Alonso, D. R., Scheidt, S., Post, M. and Killip, T.: Pathophysiology of cardiogenic shock: quantification of myocardial necrosis, clinical, pathologic and electrocardiographic correlations. *Circulation, 48,* 588, 1973.

8. Ratshin, R. A., Rackley, C. E. and Russell, R. O., Jr.: Hemodynamic evaluation of left ventricular function in shock complicating myocardial infarction. *Circulation, 45,* 127, 1972.

9. Henning, R. J. and Weil, M. H.: Effect of afterload reduction on plasma volume during acute heart failure. *Amer. J. Cardiol., 42,* 823, 1978.

10. Dawson, V. T., Harr, R. F., Hallman, G. L. and Cooley, D. A.: Mortality in patients undergoing coronary artery bypass surgery after myocardial infarction. *Amer. J. Cardiol., 33,* 483, 1974.

11. Bardet, J., Rigaud, M., Kahn, J. C., Huret, J. F., Gandjbakhch, I. and Bourdarias, J. P.: Treatment of post myocardial angina by intra-aortic balloon pumping and emergency revascularization. *J. Thoracic Cardiovasc. Surg., 74,* 299, 1977.

9

Drugs used in myocardial infarction*

> The prompt detection and treatment of arrhythmias is the principal goal of the Coronary Care Unit.

Major arrhythmias such as ventricular fibrillation and ventricular standstill often are preceded by minor arrhythmias. Drug treatment of minor arrhythmias is usually effective and thus prevents more serious arrhythmias.

THE ETIOLOGY OF ARRHYTHMIAS

> Acute myocardial infarction may affect the cardiac rhythm by:
>
> 1. Stimulating ectopic foci (facilitating reentry).
> 2. Suppressing normal foci.

*Dosage of drugs and other details may be found on pages 129–132.

Treatment of arrhythmias is directed toward altering one or both of these mechanisms, often with drugs.

ROUTE OF ADMINISTRATION OF DRUGS

> Route of administration for acute problems is INTRAVENOUS because of rapid distribution and effect.

The intravenous route, with rapid distribution and effect, is often best for the acute problem, whether pain, heart failure, shock, resuscitation, or arrhythmia. Oral medication often is vomited. Both oral and intramuscular medication are absorbed too slowly. An additional advantage of the intravenous route is the safety it allows by precise adjustment of dosage. Response may be evaluated soon after a small dose; further medication is given only if needed. In an urgent situation, repeated oral or intramuscular doses often overshoot the therapeutic level. This is especially likely if, in an emergency, an intravenous dose is given before previously-administered oral or intramuscular medication has been fully absorbed.

> All patients in the CCU should have an I.V. drip as a route for the administration of medication. Avoid using the antecubital veins, preserving these for flow-directed pressure and transvenous pacing catheters.

DRUGS USED IN TREATING ARRHYTHMIAS

Drugs Which Suppress Ectopic Foci

Drugs such as lidocaine (Xylocaine®), quinidine, procainamide (Pronestyl®), diphenylhydantoin (Dilantin) and propranolol (Inderal®) *depress* the myocardium, and consequently may suppress ectopic foci. Ectopic foci may arise in the atrium, the A-V node, or the ventricle.

> Lidocaine is the initial treatment of choice for ventricular premature contractions and ventricular tachycardia.

Lidocaine is an excellent drug with a wide range of safety. Its onset of action is within two minutes, so that it may be repeated two or three times every two or three minutes, till a response is obtained. Treatment is best initiated with an I.V. bolus of 50–100 mg., choosing the smaller dosages for smaller individuals or patients with low cardiac output or liver disease. The drug is detoxified in the liver and has a half-life of about 90 minutes. Because of equilibration between bloodstream and tissues, the antiarrhythmic effect lasts only 10 to 20 minutes after a bolus dose. To maintain an adequate blood level, a second bolus is necessary after 10 minutes. The I.V. boli should be followed with an I.V. drip. Commonly, the I.V. drip is prepared to contain 1.0 mg. per cc. and is given at a rate of 1–4 mg./min. The faster rates of I.V. drip are used in cases which required larger initial doses and in larger individuals. The dosage should be adjusted until benefit is obtained, other treatment is instituted, or toxicity occurs.

Toxic signs consist of *twitching, vague visual symptoms, dizziness, or convulsions.* Toxicity is rare below 5 mg./min. or 2–3 Gm./24 hours. Various degrees of *A-V block* have been noted with lidocaine, so it should not be given to a patient with A-V block unless a pacing catheter is in place. Once the arrhythmia is controlled with lidocaine, the I.V. drip may be slowed gradually, watching for recurrence of the arrhythmia. Generally the drip can be discontinued without "weaning" after 24 hours.

Quinidine and *Pronestyl®* have actions similar to lidocaine but with slower onset of action, longer duration, and greater toxicity. Hypotension due to intravenous Pronestyl and gastrointestinal symptoms with oral quinidine are particularly common and undesirable.

Dilantin seems to have its greatest usefulness in controlling ectopic foci due to digitalis toxicity. It is most effective intravenously but is highly irritating and prone to cause local thrombophlebitis.

Inderal®, with its tendency to aggravate heart failure and shock, has limited use in acute myocardial infarction. Recent studies suggest it may be useful for reducing myocardial ischemia, and for ventricular arrhythmias resistant to other drugs.

Bretylol® (bretylium tosylate) may be effective in ventricular arrhythmias which are resistant to first line drugs such as lidocaine or procainamide.

Drugs Used to Slow A-V Conduction

Supraventricular tachycardias such as atrial tachycardia, atrial flutter, or atrial fibrillation may be treated by slowing conduction through the A-V node. *Digitalis* is the most effective drug for this action; it reduces the number of atrial impulses passing through the A-V node, and thus slows the ventricular rate. *Inderal®* has an action on the A-V node similar to digitalis and might be used as a second choice. Occasionally, atrial or junctional tachycardias are *due to digitalis,* and in this instance digitalis is stopped and *potassium* or *Dilantin* might be used.

Drugs Used for Bradycardia or A-V Block

Acute myocardial infarction (or drugs) may suppress a normal pacemaker such as the sinus or A-V node, producing bradycardia or A-V block. Bradycardia due to suppression of the sinus node or A-V block may be followed by the *"escape"* of a lower pacemaking focus. It is the *"escape"* that prevents ventricular standstill in third degree A-V block. Treatment is aimed at increasing the heart rate, rather than abolishing the lower focus.

"Escape" arrhythmias are treated by producing a faster rhythm, using drugs or pacing.

Sinus bradycardia, and occasionally first and second degree A-V block, may respond to *atropine* since it counteracts the slowing action of the vagus nerve on the sinus and A-V nodes. Atropine occasionally may aggravate second degree A-V block since more sinus impulses will arrive at the already depressed A-V node. *Isuprel®* stimulates the sinus node and relieves sinus bradycardia. Occasionally it is used also as a *temporary measure* to stimulate the rate of an idioventricular focus in third degree A-V block, but it has the disadvantage of producing other ventricular arrhythmias by increasing myocardial excitability.

DRUGS USED IN CARDIOPULMONARY RESUSCITATION

Cardiac arrest is promptly complicated by *acidosis* due to anaerobic metabolism.

> Acidosis makes cardiac arrest more resistant to correction, causes cerebral and respiratory depression, and predisposes to arrhythmias after arrest is corrected.

Sodium bicarbonate is used to combat acidosis. Initially, during cardiac arrest, fifty ml. of 7.5% solution are given intravenously and repeated every five minutes.

Isuprel® or *epinephrine* may stimulate cardiac activity in ventricular standstill. Ideally, they should be given into the heart or via a central venous catheter if in place. Epinephrine may facilitate defibrillation if initial precordial shocks are unsuccessful.

Lidocaine is used frequently to facilitate defibrillation or prevent its recurrence.

Calcium chloride may be used to treat myocardial hypotonicity ("flabbiness") which results in poor or absent myocardial contractions.

DRUGS USED IN CONGESTIVE HEART FAILURE

> The goals of drug treatment in congestive heart failure are to:
>
> 1. Enhance the pumping action of the heart.
> 2. Increase excretion of sodium and water by the kidneys.

Digitalis is given to improve the pumping action of the heart. A "short-acting" preparation such as digoxin (Lanoxin®) is preferred. It has a rapid onset of action and is quickly excreted should toxicity occur.

Furosemide (Lasix®) and *ethacrynic acid* (Edecrin®) are potent diuretics which have a rapid onset of action. They may be given intravenously.

Thiazides such as chlorothiazide and hydrochlorothiazide are other effective diuretics. All may result in potassium depletion, alkalosis, and acute gout. Selection and dosage are dictated by the individual situation.

Vasodilators are used in congestive heart failure to reduce peripheral resistance and/or allow pooling of blood peripherally. *Nitroglycerin* and long-acting nitrates such as *isosorbide dinitrate* are primarily venous dilators resulting in venous pooling. *Hydralazine* and *prazosin* are predominately arterial dilators and hence reduce peripheral vascular resistance. Some vasodilator agents have a balanced dilating effect, improving cardiac output, reducing left ventricular filling pressure, and reducing systemic pressure. *Sodium nitroprusside* and *phentolamine* are examples of these. Vasodilators should not be used unless left ventricular filling pressure is high since a fall in cardiac output would result (review Starling's Law).

DRUGS USED FOR CHEST PAIN

Morphine and *Demerol*®, given intravenously, are the primary drugs used for control of pain of myocardial infarction.

Recent studies suggest vasodilators such as nitroglycerin and long-acting nitrates relieve pain of myocardial ischemia and may preserve myocardium. *Inderal,* through its beta-adrenergic blocking action, may also be useful in relieving myocardial ischemia.

DRUGS USED FOR HYPERTENSION

Hypertension results in increased afterload, myocardial work, and myocardial oxygen consumption. Prompt therapy is indicated. *Sodium nitroprusside* is the drug of choice because of its rapid onset of action and equally rapid clearing in case of excess dosage. Constant attention to the infusion is necessary. Therapy with other drugs such as Methyldopa (Aldomet®) or furosemide (Lasix®) may also be used in less urgent situations or as maintenance therapy.

DRUGS USED IN SHOCK

Drugs given in the treatment of shock generally are directed toward increasing the blood pressure and improving the blood flow to the vital organs such as the heart, brain, liver, and kidneys. Observation of urine output, pulmonary artery oxygen saturation, and pulmonary capillary wedge pressure often are helpful in assessing whether adequate dosage is being administered or satisfactory response is occurring. Unfortunately, none of the drugs is entirely satisfactory in its actions, as demonstrated in the following chart.

Drug	Cardiac Output	Peripheral Resistance	Renal Blood Flow
Dopamine HCl Intropin®	↓ no change or ↑ *	no change or ↑ *	↑ or ↓ *
Phenylephrine hydrochloride Neosynephrine®	↓	↑	↓
Mephentermine sulphate Wyamine®	↑	↑	↓
Norepinephrine Levophed®	↓ or no change	↑	↓
Metaraminol Aramine®	↓ or no change	↑	↓
Sodium Nitroprusside Nipride®	↑ or ↓	↑	↑ or no change

*at doses over 30 mcg./kg./min.

None of these drugs is helpful where there is a deficit in circulating blood volume. *Fluid balance* must be assessed carefully before vasopressor treatment of shock is instituted. *Respiratory exchange* must be evaluated, as poor ventilation often contributes to shock.

Sodium bicarbonate, oxygen, vasodilators, and digitalis are often used as supplementary treatment in shock.

DRUGS USED TO PREVENT THROMBOEMBOLISM

Anticoagulants prolong the clotting time of blood. Indications for their use in acute myocardial infarction include:

> 1. Reduction in the incidence of peripheral venous thrombi and subsequent pulmonary emboli.
> 2. Reduction in the formation of mural thrombi.

Two types of anticoagulants are used:

Heparin is given intravenously when an immediate anticoagulant effect is desired. Continuous infusion with an infusion pump or drop regulator after an initial bolus is preferred to intermittent I.V. or subcutaneous therapy because more constant levels are achieved. Dosage is controlled by the determination of clotting time, partial thromboplastin time, or recalcification time, aiming for a range of about twice the normal range. Heparin overdosage may be treated with *protamine sulfate* or freshly-drawn whole blood.

Coumarin derivatives (Warfarin®, Coumadin®, Dicumarol®) are slow in onset of action, requiring 5 to 7 days to depress several clotting factors. Oral administration is their principal advantage. Dosage is related to the drug selected and is controlled by measuring the *prothrombin time,* aiming for a prolongation of 2 to 2½ times the control time. Abnormal bleeding is more common with excessive dosage of coumarin derivatives than with heparin. Overdosage may be counteracted with *Vitamin K-1* (AquaMEPHYTON®), given orally or intravenously.

> Complications of anticoagulants are as follows:
>
> 1. Occult bleeding is common.
> 2. Local bleeding at injection sites may occur.
> 3. Increased sensitivity to coumarin derivatives in congestive heart failure makes control of dosage difficult.

MANAGEMENT OF MYOCARDIAL INFARCTION

Prompt professional response to reported symptoms. Trained ambulance personnel. Prompt transfer to hospital. Prompt admission to ICCF.	If symptoms suspicious enough to warrant hospitalization, immediate ICC needed.	Monitor. Start I.V. (to provide route for urgent medication). Defibrillator at bedside, ready to use. Write orders for routine and emergency measures.

CONGESTIVE HEART FAILURE?	PULMONARY EDEMA?	SHOCK?
Oxygen. Diuretics. Digoxin (I.V., fractional doses). Sodium restriction. Monitor pulmonary artery pressure or wedge pressure. Edecrin® or Lasix® I.V. Vasodilators.	Morphine I.V. Oxygen. Rotating tourniquets. Phlebotomy? Dangle. Digoxin I.V. Edecrin® or Lasix® I.V. Follow PCWP carefully.	Monitor pulmonary artery pressure or wedge pressure. If PCWP low or normal, consider fluid replacement with repeated challenge doses. Monitor hourly urine volume. Determine position which provides maximum comfort and maximum BP. Recall unreliability of BP measurements. Oxygen. Consider dopamine. Consider digoxin (especially if PCWP high). Consider Levophed® or Aramine®. Consider Vasodilators.

DIGITALIS TOXICITY?
Check serum potassium and history of potassium intake and output. Avoid precordial shock. Consider lidocaine, quinidine or Pronestyl.® Dilantin or Inderal® I.V., if ventricular arrhythmias. Pace if A-V block results in serious fall in C.O.

FIRST DEGREE A-V HEART BLOCK?	SECOND DEGREE A-V HEART BLOCK?	THIRD DEGREE A-V HEART BLOCK?
Try atropine, I.V. Avoid morphine, if possible. Hold digitalis. Prepare pacing equipment.	Atropine, I.V. Consider transvenous pacing catheter. Avoid quinidine, Pronestyl®, lidocaine, unless paced.	Avoid quindine, Pronestyl®, lidocaine, unless paced. Isuprel.® Pacing catheter and demand pulse generator. Don't hesitate to pace via percutaneous ventricular puncture if situation is urgent and transvenous catheterization not promptly successful.

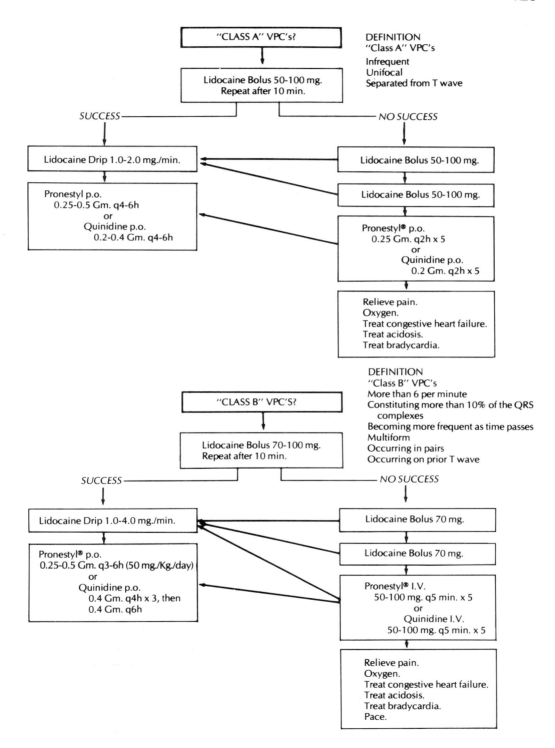

"CLASS A" VPC's?

DEFINITION
"Class A" VPC's
Infrequent
Unifocal
Separated from T wave

Lidocaine Bolus 50-100 mg.
Repeat after 10 min.

SUCCESS —————————— *NO SUCCESS*

Lidocaine Drip 1.0-2.0 mg./min.

Lidocaine Bolus 50-100 mg.

Pronestyl p.o.
0.25-0.5 Gm. q4-6h
or
Quinidine p.o.
0.2-0.4 Gm. q4-6h

Lidocaine Bolus 50-100 mg.

Pronestyl® p.o.
0.25 Gm. q2h x 5
or
Quinidine p.o.
0.2 Gm. q2h x 5

Relieve pain.
Oxygen.
Treat congestive heart failure.
Treat acidosis.
Treat bradycardia.

DEFINITION
"Class B" VPC's
More than 6 per minute
Constituting more than 10% of the QRS
complexes
Becoming more frequent as time passes
Multiform
Occurring in pairs
Occurring on prior T wave

"CLASS B" VPC'S?

Lidocaine Bolus 70-100 mg.
Repeat after 10 min.

SUCCESS —————————— *NO SUCCESS*

Lidocaine Drip 1.0-4.0 mg./min.

Lidocaine Bolus 70 mg.

Pronestyl® p.o.
0.25-0.5 Gm. q3-6h (50 mg./Kg./day)
or
Quinidine p.o.
0.4 Gm. q4h x 3, then
0.4 Gm. q6h

Lidocaine Bolus 70 mg.

Pronestyl® I.V.
50-100 mg. q5 min. x 5
or
Quinidine I.V.
50-100 mg. q5 min. x 5

Relieve pain.
Oxygen.
Treat congestive heart failure.
Treat acidosis.
Treat bradycardia.
Pace.

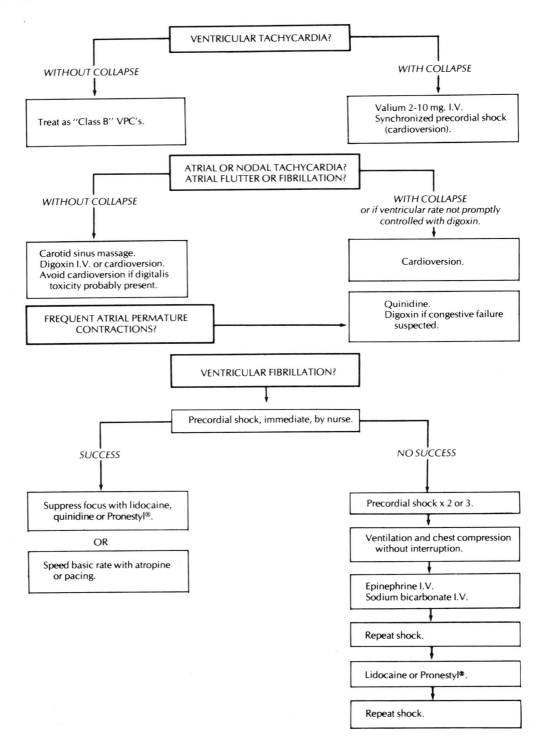

VENTRICULAR TACHYCARDIA?

WITHOUT COLLAPSE

Treat as "Class B" VPC's.

WITH COLLAPSE

Valium 2-10 mg. I.V.
Synchronized precordial shock
(cardioversion).

ATRIAL OR NODAL TACHYCARDIA?
ATRIAL FLUTTER OR FIBRILLATION?

WITHOUT COLLAPSE

WITH COLLAPSE
or if ventricular rate not promptly
controlled with digoxin.

Carotid sinus massage.
Digoxin I.V. or cardioversion.
Avoid cardioversion if digitalis
toxicity probably present.

Cardioversion.

FREQUENT ATRIAL PERMATURE
CONTRACTIONS?

Quinidine.
Digoxin if congestive failure
suspected.

VENTRICULAR FIBRILLATION?

Precordial shock, immediate, by nurse.

SUCCESS

NO SUCCESS

Suppress focus with lidocaine,
quinidine or Pronestyl®.

OR

Speed basic rate with atropine
or pacing.

Precordial shock x 2 or 3.

Ventilation and chest compression
without interruption.

Epinephrine I.V.
Sodium bicarbonate I.V.

Repeat shock.

Lidocaine or Pronestyl®.

Repeat shock.

A SUMMARY OF ARRHYTHMIAS

Rhythm	Significance	ECG	Treatment
SINUS BRADYCARDIA	Low cardiac output if stroke volume limited.	Rate less than 60. PR constant and normal.	Atropine, pacing.
SINUS TACHYCARDIA	Low cardiac output when filling time inadequate.	Rate more than 100. PR constant and normal.	Treat basic problem.
SINUS ARRHYTHMIA	Usually none.	PR constant and normal. Variable R-R interval.	None.
ATRIAL PREMATURE CONTRACTIONS	Often indicate congestive failure. May lead to other atrial arrhythmias.	Premature P with different configuration.	None, or consider quinidine or digitalis.
ATRIAL TACHYCARDIA	Cardiac output may fall. Suggests digitalis toxicity.	P often hidden. Ventricular rhythm regular. Rate about 200.	Carotid pressure, digitalis, cardioversion, Tensilon.
ATRIAL FLUTTER	Often indicates congestive failure. Cardiac output may fall.	Flutter waves, 300 per minute. Usually 2:1, 3:1, 4:1 or variable A-V conduction.	Cardioversion, digitalis.
ATRIAL FIBRILLATION	Often indicates congestive failure. Cardiac output may fall.	Fibrillation waves, 350-500/min., with variable contour.	Digitalis, cardioversion.

Rhythm	Significance	ECG	Treatment
JUNCTIONAL PREMATURE CONTRACTIONS	Same as APC's.	Ventricular rhythm irregular. Inverted P precedes, is buried in, or follows QRS.	Same as APC's.
JUNCTIONAL TACHYCARDIA	Sames as atrial tachycardia. Suggests digitalis toxicity	Inverted P precedes, is buried in, or follows, QRS.	Sames as atrial tachycardia.
VENTRICULAR PREMATURE CONTRACTIONS	May lead to ventricular tachycardia or fibrillation.	QRS premature, broad, "different" and not preceded by premature P.	Lidocaine, quinidine, Pronestyl®
VENTRICULAR TACHYCARDIA	Often progresses to vascular collapse or ventricular fibrillation.	QRS broad. Ventricular rhythm nearly regular. P unrelated to QRS. Average rate 180.	Lidocaine, quinidine, Pronestyl®, cardioversion.
VENTRICULAR FIBRILLATION	No cardiac output. Fatal if untreated.	No well-defined QRS. Irregular undulations.	Precordial shock.
FIRST DEGREE A-V BLOCK	May progress to higher degree block. May indicate excess quinidine, Pronestyl®, or digitalis.	PR 0.21 sec. or more. Each P conducted.	Observe for higher degree block.
SECOND DEGREE A-V BLOCK	May progress to complete block.	Some P waves not conducted.	Insert pacemaker catheter. Atropine.
THIRD DEGREE A-V BLOCK	Low cardiac output. May produce shock, congestive failure, syncope, ventricular arrhythmias.	P unrelated to QRS. Ventricular rate 20-45. QRS narrow or broad.	Pacemaker. Isuprel® may speed ventricular rate, but used only temporarily.

CARDIOVASCULAR DRUGS

Drug	Usual Dose	Uses	Toxicity
LANOXIN® DIGOXIN	Digitalizing dose: 2.0-3.0 mg. orally; 1.0-2.0 mg. I.V.	Congestive heart failure, control ventricular rate in atrial flutter or fibrillation.	VPC's, A-V conduction disturbances, nausea, vomiting, yellow vision, and other CNS symptoms.
DIGITOXIN	Digitalizing dose: 1.0-2.0 mg. orally.	Same as digoxin but slower action and more prolonged effect.	Same as digoxin; toxicity more prolonged.
XYLOCAINE® LIDOCAINE	70-100 mg. I.V. x 3; 1.0-4.0 mg/min. I.V. drip.	Ventricular arrhythmias.	Seizures, A-V block.
PRONESTYL® PROCAINAMIDE	0.5 Gm. q 6 h orally; 50-100 mg. I.V. q 5 min. x 5.	Atrial and ventricular arrhythmias.	Hypotension, diarrhea, intraventricular conduction delay, ventricular arrhythmias, skin rash, systemic lupus erythematosis.
QUINIDINE	0.2-0.4 Gm. q 4 h orally; 100 mg. I.V. q 5 min. x 5.	Atrial and ventricular arrhythmias.	GI symptoms, tinnitus, fever, syncope, thrombocytopenia, hypotension, intraventricular conduction delay, ventricular arrhythmias.
BRETYLOL® BRETYLIUM TOSYLATE	5 mg./kg. I.V. over 8 minute period or I.M. Increase to 10 mg./kg. at 15-30 min. intervals up to 30 mg./kg.	Ventricular tachycardia or ventricular fibrillation.	Hypotension with low dose, nausea, vomiting, bradycardia, angina.

Drug	Usual Dose	Uses	Toxicity
DILANTIN® DIPHENYLHYDANTOIN	250 mg., diluted in 5 cc. solution, I.V. slowly over 5 min.; 100 mg. q.i.d. orally.	Arrhythmias due to digitalis toxicity. Prophylactically prior to cardioversion.	Local thrombophlebitis. Respiratory arrest.
INDERAL® PROPRANOLOL	10–80 mg. q 6 h orally; 0.5–1.0 mg./min. I.V.	Atrial and ventricular arrhythmias, angina.	Heart failure, shock, asthma, A-V block.
ATROPINE	0.5–1.0 mg./min. I.V.	Sinus bradycardia, A-V block.	May slow ventricular rate in 2° A-V block, glaucoma, urinary retention, delirium, fever.
ISUPREL® ISOPROTERENOL	0.2–1.0 mg. in 500 cc. I.V. drip.	Bradycardia, third degree A-V block.	Tachycardia, ventricular arrhythmias, myocardial necrosis.
EPINEPHRINE	1.0 mg. (1 cc. of 1:1000) I.V.	Ventricular fibrillation when no response to precordial shock.	Tachycardia, ventricular arrhythmias.
SODIUM BICARBONATE, 7.5%	50 cc. initially, repeated every 5 min. of circulatory arrest.	Correction of accidosis due to circulatory arrest or shock.	Local thrombophlebitis, sodium excess.

Drug	Usual Dose	Uses	Toxicity
EDECRIN® ETHACRYNIC ACID	25–50 mg. I.V., 50–400 mg. orally in divided doses.	Acute pulmonary edema, congestive heart failure, hypertension.	Potassium depletion, alkalosis, excess diuresis, acute gout, thrombocytopenia.
LASIX® FUROSEMIDE	10–80 mg. I.V.; 40–320 mg. orally.	Same as ethacrynic acid.	Potassium depletion, alkalosis, excess diuresis.
INTROPIN® DOPAMINE HCl	2–5 mcg./kg./min. initially, increase q 10 min. to desired effect. Dosage over 30 mcg./kg./min. acts like norepinephrine.	Shock, chronic congestive heart failure.	Ectopic beats, nausea, vomiting, tachycardia, angina.
GLUCAGON	2.5–5.0 mg. I.V. infusion, 1–4 mcg./kg./min.	Shock, acute heart failure, especially where propranolol has been used.	Nausea, hypoglycemia, hypokalemia.
ARAMINE® METARAMINOL	50–200 mg./L; give 2–3 cc./min. I.V.	Shock.	Uses body's own catecholamines so may need increasing dose, ventricular arrhythmias, excessive vasopressor response persists 20–60 min.
LEVOPHED® NOREPINEPHRINE	1–4 ampules (4–16 mg. Levophed base) per liter, 20–30 drops per min.	Shock.	Cutaneous necrosis (treat with Regitine), reduction of blood volume, ventricular arrhythmias.
WYAMINE® MEPHENTERMINE	1000 mg./L.; give 1-3 cc./min.	Shock.	CNS stimulation.

Drug	Usual Dose	Uses	Toxicity
NIPRIDE® SODIUM NITROPRUSSIDE	0.5–8 mcg./kg./min. Must be protected from light and not kept or used over 4 hours.	Hypertension, congestive heart failure.	Nausea, sweating, headache, angina, palpitation.
ALDOMET® METHYLDOPA	250–500 mg. q 6–8 hr. I.V. or PO.	Hypertension.	Somnolence, Parkinsonism.
APRESOLINE® HYDRALAZINE	25–100 mg. PO q 6 h.	Hypertension, congestive heart failure.	Postural hypotension, peripheral neuritis, blood dyscrasias, lupus erythematosis.
NITROGLYCERIN	Tablet—.3–.6 mg. sublingually 2–3 times. I.V.—8–80 mcg./min., average 30 mg./min. Paste—½–2 inches q 4–6 hr.	Angina, congestive heart failure.	Headache, tachycardia, hypotension.
ISORDIL® SORBITRATE® ISOSORBIDE DINITRATE	2.5–10 mg. q 4–6 hr.	Angina, congestive heart failure.	Headache, tachycardia, hypotension, nausea, vomiting.
MINIPRESS® PRAZOSIN HCl	1–5 mg. q 8 hr. PO.	Hypertension, congestive heart failure.	Hypotension, nausea, vomiting, fluid retention.
HEPARIN	5000–15,000 units I.V.; 10,000–20,000 units subcutaneously.	Decrease blood clotting tendency, prevent thrombi and emboli; control dose with clotting time.	Bleeding. Antidote: protamine sulfate or fresh blood.
COUMADIN® PANWARFIN® WARFARIN SODIUM	30–60 mg. initially, 2–10 mg. daily.	Same as heparin. Control dose with prothrombin time.	Bleeding. Antidote: Vitamin K (Mephyton®).

COMMON SIGNS OF DRUG TOXICITY

Drug	Reason For Use	Reasons For Nurse to Withhold Dose Until Physician is Notified
DIGITALIS	To strengthen contraction. To reduce A-V conduction.	Vomiting. VPC's or other new arrhythmia. Bradycardia.
LIDOCAINE	To suppress VPC's.	Twitching. Convulsion. A-V block.
QUINIDINE or PRONESTYL®	To suppress ectopic foci.	Fall in BP. Diarrhea. Prolongation of PR or QRS.
ISUPREL®	To speed rate of sinus node or idioventricular pacemaker.	Ventricular arrhythmias.
ANTICOAGULANTS	To prevent mural or venous thrombus.	Bleeding. Excessive clotting time or prothrombin time.

QUESTIONS—CHAPTER 9

1. The best route for administration of drugs for an acute problem is _____

   intravenous.

---

2. Every patient in the CCU should have an I.V. drip:

   A. ____ To maintain fluid balance.

   B. ____ As a route for the administration of medication.

   C. ____ To facilitate the measurement of central venous pressure.

   B

---

3. For the treatment of severe pain or an arrhythmia, the intravenous route of drug administration is preferred because it:

   A. _____

   _____

   Provides rapid action.

   B. _____

   _____

   Avoids variable absorption of oral and I.M. medications.

   C. _____

   _____

   Allows precise adjustment of dosage.

4. Acute myocardial infarction may affect the cardiac rhythm by:

    A. _____ Suppressing normal foci.   *A*

    B. _____ Stimulating normal foci.

    C. _____ Stimulating abnormal foci.   *C*

    D. _____ Suppressing abnormal foci.

5. Arrhythmias due to ectopic foci are treated by:

    A. _____ Suppressing the ectopic foci.   *A*

    B. _____ Digitalis.   *B*

    C. _____ Lidocaine.   *C*

    D. _____ Slowing A-V conduction.   *D*

    E. _____ Increasing the heart rate.   *E*

    F. _____ Treating acidosis with sodium bicarbonate.

6. Drugs such as lidocaine, quinidine, Pronestyl®, Dilantin, and Inderal® _____ the myocardium.   *depress*

7. Lidocaine is the treatment of choice for:

    A. _____   *Ventricular premature contractions.*

    B. _____   *Ventricular tachycardia.*

8. Slow rhythms such as sinus bradycardia and A-V block may respond to drugs which _____ normal pacemaker sites.   *stimulate*

9. Escape arrhythmias are treated by producing a _____ rate.	*faster*
10. Atropine stimulates the sinus node by _____ .	*counteracting the slowing action of the vagus nerve.*
11. Third degree A-V block should be treated with:	
A. ____ Isuprel®.	
B. ____ Atropine.	
C. ____ Pacing.	*C*
D. ____ Lidocaine.	
E. ____ Corticosteroids.	
12. In cardiac arrest, acidosis:	
A. ____ Predisposes to arrhythmias after correction of arrest.	*A*
B. ____ Stimulates the myocardium.	
C. ____ Depresses the respiratory center.	*C*
D. ____ Makes the arrest less responsive to correction.	*D*

13. The goals of drug treatment of congestive heart failure are to:

    A. _____

        _____

        Improve the pumping action of the heart.

    B. _____

        _____

        Increase excretion of sodium and water.

14. A drug which usually is effective in severe cardiogenic shock is:

    A. ____ Levophed®.

    B. ____ Isuprel®.

    C. ____ Yet to be discovered.   *C*

    D. ____ Dopamine.

15. Guides to treating shock include:

    A. ____ Urine output.   *A*

    B. ____ Central venous pressure.   *B*

    C. ____ Assessment of respiratory exchange.   *C*

    D. ____ Evaluation of fluid balance.   *D*

    E. ____ Determination of blood volume.   *E*

    F. ____ Pulmonary artery diastolic pressure.   *F*

16. In acute myocardial infarction, anticoagulants are used to:

    A. _____

       _____

    Reduce peripheral venous thrombi and pulmonary emboli.

    B. _____

       _____

    Reduce the formation of mural thrombi and subsequent peripheral emboli.

---

17. Match the action of digitalis with the clinical problem:

    A. ____ Strengthens myocardial contraction.

    2, 3

    B. ____ Slows conduction through the A-V node.

    1, 4

    1. Atrial fibrillation.

    2. Shock.

    3. Congestive heart failure.

    4. Atrial tachycardia.

---

18. Atropine might be used to treat sinus bradycardia. What other drug might be used?

    _____

    Isuprel®, but serious ventricular arrhythmias frequently occur. Pacing is the treatment of choice in symptomatic sinus bradycardia

19. Third degree A-V block should be treated with:

    A. _____ Isuprel®.

    B. _____ Atropine.

    C. _____ Transvenous pacing.   C

---

20. Ventricular fibrillation may not respond to precordial shock if the myocardium is depressed by anoxia and acidosis. What drug might improve myocardial tone and responsiveness to precordial shock?

    _____   *Epinephrine*

---

21. Match the anticoagulant with the properties below:

    A. _____ Heparin.   *1, 4*

    B. _____ Coumarin derivatives.   *2, 3*

    1. Rapid onset of action.

    2. Oral administration.

    3. Dose determined by prothrombin time.

    4. Dose determined by clotting time.

22. Indicate the drugs often used in treatment of these arrhythmias:

A. _____ Atrial flutter.   *2, 5*

B. _____ Ventricular premature con-   *1, 3, 5*
         tractions.

C. _____ Atrial fibrillation.   *2, 5*

D. _____ Second degree A-V block.   *7*

E. _____ Atrial premature contractions.   *2, 5*

F. _____ Ventricular tachycardia.   *1, 3, 5*

G. _____ Ventricular standstill.   *4, 6*

H. _____ Sinus bradycardia.   *7*

1. Lidocaine

2. Digitalis

3. Pronestyl®

4. Isuprel®

5. Quinidine

6. Epinephrine

7. Atropine

SUGGESTED READING — CHAPTER 9

1.   Wyman, M. G., Lalka, D., Hammersmith, L., Cannon, D. S. and Goldreyer, B. N.: Multiple bolus technique for lidocaine administration during the first hours of an acute myocardial infarction. *Amer. J. Cardiol., 41,* 313, 1978.

2.   Wyman, M. G. and Hammersmith, L.: Comprehensive treatment plan for the prevention of primary ventricular fibrillation in acute myocardial infarction. *Amer. J. Cardiol., 33,* 661, 1974.

3.   Gazes, P. C. and Gaddy, J. E.: Bedside management of acute myocardial infarction. *Amer. Heart J., 97,* 782, 1979.

4.   Armstrong, P. W., Walker, D. C., Burton, J. R. and Parker, J. O.: Vasodilator therapy in acute myocardial infarction. A comparison of sodium nitroprusside and nitroglycerine. *Circulation, 52,* 1118, 1975.

5.   Rahimtoola, S. H.: Digitalis in acute myocardial infarction: help or hazard? *Ann. Intern. Med., 82,* 234, 1975.

6.   Mantle, J. A., Russell, R. O., Jr., Moraski, R. E. and Rackley, C. E.: Isosorbide dinitrate for the relief of severe heart failure after myocardial infarction. *Amer. J. Cardiol., 37,* 263, 1976.

7.   Winkle, R. A., Glantz, S. A. and Harrison, D. C.: Pharmacological therapy of ventricular arrhythmias. *Amer. J. Cardio., 36,* 629, 1975.

8.   Lima, J. J., Goldfarb, A. L., Conti, D. R., Golden, L. H., Bascomb, B. L., Benedetti, G. M. and Jusko, W. J.: Safety and efficacy of procainamide infusions. *Amer. J. Cardiol., 43,* 98, 1979.

9.   Stemple, D. R., Kleiman, J. H. and Harrison, D. C.: Combined nitroprusside-dopamine therapy in severe chronic congestive heart failure. Dose-related hemodynamic advantages over single drug infusions. *Amer. J. Cardiol., 42,* 267, 1978.

10. Harrison, D. C.: Should lidocaine be administered routinely to all patients after acute myocardial infarction? *Circulation, 58,* 581, 1978.

11. Rogers, W. J., Segall, P. H., McDaniel, H. G., Mantle, J. A., Russell, R. O., Jr. and Rackley, C. E.: Prospective randomized trial of glucose-insulin-potassium in acute myocardial infarction. *Amer. J. Cardiol., 43,* 801, 1979.

12. Marcus, F. I.: Current concepts of digoxin therapy. *Mod. Concepts Cardiovasc. Dis., 45,* 77, 1976.

13. Atkinson, A. J., Jr.: Clinical use of blood levels of cardiac drugs. *Mod. Concepts Cardiovasc. Dis., 42,* 1, 1973.

10

Cardiac arrest

> The absence of effective circulation is termed cardiac arrest.

RECOGNITION OF CARDIAC ARREST

Loss of consciousness, within a few seconds.

Absence of carotid or femoral pulse. In the CCU, the monitor will show ventricular fibrillation or ventricular standstill. Either pattern plus sudden unconsciousness are adequate for the diagnosis.

Absence of respirations. Initially, respirations are usually gaspy but generally cease entirely in 30 to 60 seconds.

Some signs are *unreliable* for recognition of cardiac arrest. The *pupils* have been noted to remain constricted for one to six minutes after arrest, possibly because of prior use of drugs such as morphine. *Pulses of smaller arteries* such as the radial pulse and *auscultation* may be unreliable. Finally, the *alarm* of the monitoring system may activate for reasons other than cardiac arrest.

Cardiac arrest may be due to

1. Ventricular fibrillation
2. Ventricular standstill
3. Cardiovascular collapse

The sooner definitive treatment can be given for cardiac arrest, the greater the chances of success. In the CCU, definitive treatment is given initially, and CPR is used only if initial therapy is unsuccessful.

Ventricular Fibrillation

Ventricular fibrillation is the most common cause of cardiac arrest in patients with acute myocardial infarction.

In ventricular fibrillation, individual myocardial fibers twitch, but there is no effective ventricular contraction and no cardiac output. Without treatment, death soon results.

Time Limit

A 4-minute time limit is often referred to as the usual period of reversibility for cardiac arrest. However, *the chances of success diminish as time elapses, even during the first four minutes.* If treated in the first 30 seconds, ventricular fibrillation can almost always be reverted. If treatment is delayed only a minute or two, the success rate falls substantially.

VENTRICULAR FIBRILLATION

Primary ventricular fibrillation is the term used to describe the arrhythmia occurring without antecedent shock or heart failure. Primary ventricular fibrillation is often preceded by signs of ventricular excitability such as ventricular premature contractions or ventricular tachycardia or as an escape rhythm in heart block. Prevention of primary ventricular fibrillation is accomplished by treating the premonitory arrhythmias which precede it. Should primary ventricular fibrillation occur in the CCU, its mortality rate should be low because of prompt recognition and treatment. In general wards, recognition and treatment are both delayed and the mortality rate is high.

Secondary ventricular fibrillation describes this arrhythmia occurring secondary to profound shock or heart failure. Under these circumstances, ventricular fibrillation usually is fatal despite treatment; damage to the heart as a pump and hypoxia prevent successful treatment of this arrhythmia. Prevention of secondary ventricular fibrillation depends upon successful treatment of shock and heart failure. Little hope is yet available for these complications in myocardial infarction.

Precordial shock is the specific treatment for ventricular fibrillation. The sooner precordial shock is administered, the greater the likelihood of success.

If the first shock does not terminate fibrillation, a second or third shock may be given. By this time several minutes will have passed; since there is no circulation of blood during ventricular fibrillation, *hypoxia* and *acidosis* will develop, making the heart less responsive to defibrillation. *Hypoxia* is treated with artificial respiration and external cardiac compression. *Acidosis* is treated by the intravenous administration of sodium bicarbonate solution. Epinephrine may be administered to increase the responsiveness of the heart to precordial shock.

Standing orders, approved by the hospital staff, allow the nurse to begin appropriate therapy without delay.

STANDING ORDERS FOR VENTRICULAR FIBRILLATION

General Outline:

1. PRECORDIAL SHOCK
2. SODIUM BICARBONATE
3. SHOCK
4. EPINEPHRINE
5. SHOCK
6. LIDOCAINE
7. SHOCK

8. SHOCK
9. PRONESTYL®
10. SHOCK
11. BRETYLOL®
12. DOPAMINE or LEVOPHED
13. CALCIUM CHLORIDE
14. SHOCK

Standing Orders for Apparent Death Associated with Ventricular Fibrillation

In the event of apparent death associated with ventricular fibrillation, the nurse may undertake the following actions. This program is interrupted when effective circulation resumes.

1. Give *precordial shock* at maximum setting. Repeat several times if necessary. Often it is possible to summon aid and activate the timing clock without delaying precordial shock. A thump on the precordium may be used if, for some reason, it can be applied more promptly than precordial shock and if it will not delay this definitive treatment.

2. If fibrillation persists, *respiration and chest compression* are needed hereafter. Interrupt no more than 5 seconds every 3 minutes to carry out the following measures. CPR is more important than drugs.

3. Start *7.5% sodium bicarbonate* 1 to 2 50cc. ampules (44.6 mEq./ampule) or 1 mEq./kg. initially, then 50 cc. during each 5 minutes that ineffective circulation continues. Check arterial blood gases as a guide.

4. Repeat *shock* 2 or 3 times.

5. If assistance has not yet arrived, rapidly inject 1 cc. 1:1000 *epinephrine* (1.0 mg.) if I.V. is running. Repeat epinephrine q 3 minutes p.r.n. times 2.

6. Precordial *shock*.

7. Rapidly inject 7 cc. 1% *lidocaine* (70 mg.) I.V.

8. Continue *chest compression and ventilation* until a physician's orders are obtained.

The P's of Precordial Shock

Electrical defibrillation is commonly performed with an external direct current defibrillator. A high-voltage shock, 6000 to 8000 volts, is delivered over a brief period of 2 to 10 milliseconds. External defibrillation is made more effective by attention to several factors.

Position

> The paddles should be positioned so that the flow of current from one paddle to the other is directed across the ventricular muscle. One electrode should be placed high on the right chest, adjacent to the sternum and below the clavicle. The other electrode is placed on the left lateral chest near the cardiac apex. Avoid placing the paddles close to a monitoring electrode.

Paste

> A "gritty" electrode paste or saline-soaked pads are applied to the electrodes to reduce skin resistance and enhance contact. Be generous, but for reasons of electrical safety, don't smear paste on your hands or the electrode handles. Don't use an electrode cream.

Pressure

> Firm pressure should be applied to the electrodes to insure good contact and reduce resistance. Avoid pressure at one edge of the paddle since it may produce contact in only a small area.

Power

> The energy discharge of the direct current defibrillator is measured in watt-seconds (joules). Though electrical defibrillation may be accomplished with a low amount of energy in some patients, it is wise to use the maximum energy delivered by the defibrillator, usually 400 watt-seconds.

Paddles

> The defibrillator electrodes should be kept polished since repeated discharge produces oxidation on the surface, increasing resistance.

Performance

> Some failures in defibrillation have been recognized as due to mechanical malfunction of the defibrillator. Recently, devices for testing defibrillators have been developed, and periodic determination of the defibrillator's performance is recommended. Ideally, there should be a defibrillator at each bedside in the CCU.

SUMMARY OF STEPS INVOLVED IN DEFIBRILLATION

1. Recognize the diagnosis from the ECG monitor pattern plus sudden unconsciousness.
2. Apply the paddles with paste, proper position, and pressure.
3. Shock, using at least 400 watt-seconds.
4. Provide other CPR measures if necessary.

VENTRICULAR STANDSTILL

Ventricular standstill is usually preceded by progressive hypoxia. It may occur if the atria cease beating or if atrial impulses are not conducted to the ventricles *and* a lower focus in the A-V node or ventricle does not arise. Standstill may result from drugs such as quinidine or excessive potassium. Failure of conduction of atrial impulses (third degree A-V block) may be due to myocardial damage or toxicity due to drugs.

During ventricular standstill, the electrocardiogram may demonstrate either no evidence of electrical activity or regularly occurring P waves without QRS complexes.

In many cases of ventricular standstill, no precipitating factor is apparent. In these "primary" situations, prompt treatment often is successful. When ventricular standstill is the result of prolonged shock or pulmonary edema or "secondary" to other profound disturbances, it represents the terminal event; treatment is ineffective.

When a patient suffers sudden, unexpected ventricular standstill, the nurse's first step in treatment is a *vigorous blow to the precordium*. If this is ineffective in restoring the circulation within a few seconds, an *internal pacemaker* should be used.

Increasing degrees of A-V block warn of the possibility of ventricular standstill. As a precautionary measure, the physician may insert a transvenous pacing catheter at the first sign of A-V conduction disorder. This permits prompt ventricular pacing, should ventricular standstill or complete (third degree) A-V block occur.

Treatment for ventricular standstill must begin immediately to be effective.

Standing Orders for Ventricular Standstill

General Outline:

1. VIGOROUS BLOW TO PRECORDIUM . . . . If unsuccessful,
   proceed to—
2. PACEMAKER . . . . If unsuccessful,
   proceed to—
3. SUMMON AID . . . .
   proceed to—
4. RESPIRATION & CHEST COMPRESSION . . . . If unsuccessful,
   proceed to—
5. ATROPINE . . . . If unsuccessful,
   proceed to—
6. ISUPREL® . . . . If unsuccessful,
   proceed to—
7. SODIUM BICARBONATE
8. CALCIUM CHLORIDE

In the event of apparent death associated with ventricular standstill, the nurse may undertake the following actions. This program is interrupted whenever effective circulation resumes.

Standing Orders for Apparent Death Associated with Ventricular Standstill

1. Give a *vigorous blow* to the precordium two or three times.
2. Use internal *pacemaker*.
   a. *Transvenous*. A transvenous pacing catheter may have been placed as a precaution.
      i) If on demand mode, as per doctor's previous orders, it should be operative already, demonstrated by a pacer blip on the oscilloscope.
      ii) If not on demand, activate at a rate of 80 per minute, using adequate voltage for ventricular response ("capture").
   b. *Transventricular*. If a pacing catheter is not in place, cardiopulmonary resuscitation must be started immediately and continued until cardiac rhythm and function are restored or a transventricular pacing catheter is placed by the physician (see Chapter 12, page 183 and Chapter 15, page 227).

3. *Summon aid* and activate timing clock.

4. *Artificial ventilation and chest compression* are needed if initial therapy is not effective in producing a palpable pulse during the first minute.

5. If there is no palpable pulse with the pacemaker and if assistance has not yet arrived, briefly interrupt respiration and compression and give *atropine,* 1.0 mg. into I.V. tubing. If there is no I.V. tubing, don't waste time trying to place one until help arrives.

6. If there is no palpable pulse, continue compression and ventilation and also give *Isuprel®* infusion, using standard solution containing 1.0 mg. Isuprel® in 500 cc. 5% glucose in water at an initial rate of 30 drops a minute.

7. If there has been no palpable pulse for three minutes, give 7.5% *sodium bicarbonate* 1 to 2 50 cc. ampules (44.6 m Eq./ampule) or 1 mEq./kg. initially, then 50 cc. during each 5 minutes that asystole continues, up to a maximum of 500 cc. Check arterial blood gases as a guide.

8. *Calcium chloride.* Give 10 cc. of 10% solution if electrical activity is present without palpable pulse.

9. If there is no palpable pulse, *continue chest compression and ventilation* until a physician's orders are obtained.

CARDIOVASCULAR COLLAPSE

Cardiovascular collapse is present when there is a coordinated electrical activity, often slow, without effective myocardial contraction. It is sometimes called "power failure." This condition often precedes ventricular standstill. It is usually due to severe myocardial hypoxia and is often an end-stage phenomenon. It may occur with anaphylaxis, hypovolemia, hypokalemia, and drug toxicity (digitalis, quinidine, procainamide).

Cardiovascular collapse is treated with cardiopulmonary resuscitation, sodium bicarbonate for acidosis, and cardiotonic drugs such as epinephrine, dopamine, and calcium chloride. Treatment is also directed to the underlying cause, if known.

CARDIOPULMONARY RESUSCITATION

There are many manuals and teaching aids available for teaching and learning the proper technique of cardiopulmonary resuscitation. A few of these include:

Emergency Measures in Cardiopulmonary Resuscitation,
American Heart Association

Definitive Therapy in Cardiopulmonary Resuscitation,
American Heart Association

The Nurse's Role in Cardiopulmonary Resuscitation,
American Heart Association

Can You Save a Life with Cardiopulmonary Resuscitation?,
Wyeth Company

Cardiopulmonary Resuscitation Conference Proceedings, 1967,
National Research Council

Each hospital and coronary care unit must have a *plan of action* for CPR since all have varying specific situations and problems which must be considered.

Once a plan of action has been developed by representatives of the physicians, nurses, and administration, the staff must be *trained, and must practice their specific duties.* Drills provide excellent preparation for future cardiac arrests.

The two factors which contribute most to the success of CPR in a hospital are:

1. The organization of equipment and personnel.
2. The training of the personnel.

STEPS IN CARDIOPULMONARY RESUSCITATION

Step	Equipment Needed
Airway	You
Breathing	You
Circulation	You
Definitive therapy	Drugs, ECG, defibrillator, pacemaker

Airway

The initial step in CPR is establishment of the airway. Actually, the initial step includes three procedures which can be started almost simultaneously:

1. *Vigorous blow to the precordium.* Occasionally this may terminate ventricular standstill and solve the entire problem.
2. *Call for help.*
3. *Establish airway.*

An open airway is best achieved by tilting the head backward.

Lifting the jaw may also help open the airway but is of less importance than tilting the head back.

Any foreign material should be removed from the mouth and throat.

Mouth-to-mouth ventilation and external cardiac compression should be started immediately. *Only after these are initiated* should one begin to think of *airway equipment.* Never wait for a gadget.

Airway Equipment:

Flanged tube with bite block ("Rescue Breather," available from Medical Supply Company, 1027 West State Street, Rockford, Illinois). This device provides hygiene, esthetics, and a good seal without problems of retching and laryngospasm in the patient. Experienced rescuers using 5 different airway devices had the *least delay* and *best tidal volume* with this one.

Oropharyngeal tube (the usual black airway). This device will lift the base of the tongue and prevent obstruction by the lips and tongue. It also produces retching and laryngospasm and is sometimes more difficult to introduce.

Oropharyngeal S-tube. This gadget has the advantages of the flanged tube and the disadvantages of the oropharyngeal tube. Its use has been overemphasized. We think it should not be used.

Oropharyngeal S-tube plus valve (Brook airway). This device has the disadvantages of the S-tube plus the problem of valve obstruction.

Bag and mask. Disadvantage of poor seal with poor tidal volume. We depart from standard teaching and advise you to forget about using a bag and mask as the initial ventilatory measure. Even nurses and doctors who have had much experience often lose precious minutes trying to get a good face seal and compress the bag simultaneously.

If the mask is used, we prefer using two hands to hold the mask to the face, tilting the head backward, then blowing into mask orifice.

> The best airway device during the emergency phase is the flanged tube with bite block.

Once the patient is well oxygenated by assisted ventilation and external cardiac compression, a *cuffed endotracheal tube* or *esophageal airway* can be considered. An esophageal airway is much easier to introduce than an endotracheal tube. **Caution:** it should not be attempted by anyone without experience or if it cannot be introduced within 30 seconds.

> Tracheal intubation is desirable since it minimizes the dangers of regurgitation, avoids gastric distention, and facilitates the use of a bag for breathing.

Breathing

Mouth-to-mouth breathing is the best way to provide ventilation during the emergency phase. Once additional assistance is obtained, an experienced rescuer may elect to use a *bag and mask.* Ventilation is poor at best, since cardiac arrest, heart failure, shock, and aspiration result in atelectasis and veno-arterial shunting.

> A bag and mask or an endotracheal tube allows the addition of oxygen to the ventilation system.

> The best breathing adjunct is an endotracheal tube plus a bag with an oxygen reservoir of at least 500 ml. Use a high oxygen flow rate of 15 L/min.

Ordinary pressure-cycled intermittent positive pressure breathing (IPPB) is *not helpful* in cardiopulmonary resuscitation because:

1. External cardiac compression triggers cessation of the inspiratory phase.
2. The flow rate is too slow to give adequate ventilation without an excessively long pause.

However, certain volume-cycled apparatus may be of use after the emergency phase; this will require careful evaluation of your equipment.

Circulation

Proper technique of external cardiac compression is essential. Even when performed perfectly, cardiac compression produces a blood flow which is only *30%* of the normal cardiac output.

The *best rate* is about *80 compressions per minute* which is difficult to sustain for an extended period.

The circulation of oxygenated blood requires both effective external cardiac compression and artificial ventilation. Excessive interruption is probably the most common cause of poor technique. External cardiac compression should never be interrupted for longer than 5 seconds.

Effectiveness of external cardiac compression is best evaluated by detection of a carotid or femoral pulse.

Other signs of both effective compression and ventilation with flow of oxygenated blood include:

1. Maintenance of normal pupil size.
2. Improvement in skin color.
3. Appearance of spontaneous respiration and movements.

Complications of external cardiac compression are minimized by proper technique, but are preferred to no resuscitation at all. Common are fractured ribs, separated costochondral junctions, and a fractured sternum. Rarely, pneumothorax or injury to the heart, the liver, or the spleen may occur.

> Use only the heel of the hand on the lower third of the sternum to avoid fractures and other injury.

DEFINITIVE THERAPY

Definitive therapy of cardiac arrest is directed toward the *cause* of the cardiac arrest and its *effects*.

Causes of Cardiac Arrest and Their Treatment

(See also Chapter 6)

Ventricular fibrillation: defibrillate with precordial shock with maximum voltage. If defibrillation is unsuccessful or fibrillation recurs:

1. Ventilation and circulation may not be adequate.
2. Acidosis may be present.
3. Drugs may be needed. Use epinephrine for fine fibrillation, lidocaine for recurrence.

Ventricular standstill: use cardiopulmonary resuscitation until an internal pacer can be placed by transthoracic puncture (see Chapter 12.)

Cardiovascular collapse (power failure): use cardiopulmonary resuscitation. Treat *effects* and underlying cause, if known.

Effects of Cardiac Arrest and Their Treatment

Acidosis: treat with 7.5% sodium bicarbonate, 50 cc. (44.6 mEq) for every 5 minutes of arrest. Err on the side of giving more than you think necessary. Check arterial blood gases after 3 ampules.

Myocardial Hypotonicity and Vasodilation: treat with epinephrine, 1.0 mg. every 5 minutes, dopamine or Levophed and calcium chloride, 1.0 Gm.

Hypoxia: treat with adequate assisted breathing and external cardiac massage.

> Do not interrupt cardiopulmonary resuscitation for more than 5 seconds to give definitive therapy.

When to Discontinue Resuscitation

1. *Cardiac Death*
   a. No electrical activity for 30 minutes.
   b. Inability to maintain satisfactory rhythm.
   c. Persistent ventricular fibrillation despite all forms of therapy.
2. *Brain Death*
   a. Fixed dilated pupils.
   b. Absence of spontaneous respiration.
3. *Patient's History*
   a. Known delay of 10 minutes or more before resuscitation began.
   b. Irreversible or terminal disease with no chance of return to functional existence.
4. No improvement of any kind after 60 minutes of intensive resuscitation.

Nurse's Responsibility in Post-Resuscitation Care

1. Monitor ECG, treat arrhythmias as ordered.
2. Monitor vital signs and neurologic status.
3. Record accurate intake and output.
4. Support ventilation and circulation as required.

Remember:

1. *Develop a plan of action* for cardiac arrest in your hospital.
2. *Definitive treatment* is the initial step in the CCU. CPR is used if initial therapy is ineffective.
3. *Train, practice, re-train.* Evaluate each instance of CPR after the crisis to improve team action.
4. *Mouth-to-mouth breathing* is the most efficient method for emergency ventilation. Ventilation devices should be simple.
5. *Tilt* the head backwards.
6. *Insert an endotracheal tube* only when personnel are available who can do so with only brief interruption of CPR. An esophageal airway is often easier to introduce.
7. *External cardiac compression* provides a cardiac output of only 30% of normal. Internal cardiac compression is no more effective than external compression and adds the risk of thoracotomy to an already desperate situation.
8. *Interrupt* ventilation or cardiac compression for no longer than 5 seconds for any reason.
9. Use only the *heel of the hand* on the lower third of the sternum.
10. Treat *acidosis* vigorously with sodium bicarbonate.
11. Treat the *specific cause* and the *effects* of cardiac arrest.

QUESTIONS—CHAPTER 10

1. The two factors which contribute most to effective cardiopulmonary resuscitation in the hospital are:

   A. _____   *Organization of equipment and personnel.*

   _____

   B. _____   *Training of the personnel.*

   _____

2. Reliable signs of cardiac arrest include:

   A. ____ Absence of respirations.   *A*

   B. ____ Constriction of the pupils.

   C. ____ Absence of carotid or femoral pulse.   *C*

   D. ____ Loss of consciousness.   *D*

   E. ____ Dilation of the pupils.

   F. ____ Activation of the alarm.

3. If not treated within 4 minutes, cardiac arrest may result in brain damage. However ventricular fibrillation and ventricular standstill respond to treatment most often within

   _____   *the first minute.*

4. When the CCU patient suddenly appears dead and the oscilloscope indicates ventricular fibrillation, the first nursing procedure is:

    A. _____ Mouth-to-mouth respiration.

    B. _____ Summon aid.

    C. _____ Notify the CCU physician on call.

    D. _____ Thump the precordium.

    E. _____ Defibrillation.

    F. _____ Intravenous epinephrine.

    G. _____ Attach pacemaker.

    H. _____ Closed chest cardiac compression.

    E

5. When ventricular fibrillation occurs on the general medical ward, mouth-to-mouth breathing and closed-chest cardiac compression maintain oxygenation of the brain and heart until definitive measures are available. In the CCU, the definitive measure is readily available and consists of _____.

    defibrillation (precordial shock).

6. If ventricular fibrillation is not reversed in the first few moments, acidosis and hypoxia develop. Since the heart's responsiveness to defibrillation is decreased by anoxia and acidosis, what measures should be carried out to treat these complications?

    A. _____

    B. _____

    C. _____

    A. Artificial respiration.

    B. Closed chest compression.

    C. I.V. sodium bicarbonate.

7. Intravenous or intracardiac epinephrine, 1.0 mg. (1.0 cc. of 1:1000 solution), is used in the treatment of ventricular fibrillation because _____ _____ _____	*it makes the heart more responsive to precordial shock.*
8. Ventricular fibrillation is accompanied by anoxia and acidosis because of the absence of circulation. Sodium bicarbonate: A. ____ Cures anoxia. B. ____ Decreases acidosis. The dose of 7.5% sodium bicarbonate is _____	*B.* *1 mEq/kg. initially (1 to 2 50 cc. ampule), then 50 cc for each 5 minutes of ineffective circulation.*
9. Mouth-to-mouth respiration gets oxygen to the lungs. External cardiac compression is necessary to: A. ____ Pump oxygenated blood to the heart and brain. B. ____ Restore the heart beat. C. ____ Get more air out of the lungs.	*A*
10. The first step in the treatment of ventricular standstill is _____ If this does not restore circulation within a few seconds, the next step is: A. ____ Precordial shock. B. ____ Activate the pacemaker.	*a vigorous blow to the precordium.* *B*

11. If a physician suspects that ventricular standstill may occur, he may insert a transvenous pacing catheter. Which of the following arrhythmias might prompt the physician to do this as a safety measure?

   A. _____ Increasing PR interval.

   A

   B. _____ Episodes of atrial fibrillation.

   C. _____ Multifocal VPC's.

   D. _____ Sinus rhythm with 2:1 A-V block.

   D

---

12. What are the first two duties when ventricular standstill develops?

   A. _____

   A. Summon aid.

   B. _____

   B. Thump the precordium.

---

13. There is no response to the above. The nurse should now:

   A. _____ Give Isuprel® I.V.

   B. _____ Give intracardiac epinephrine.

   C. _____ Begin ventilation and chest compression.

   C

   D. _____ Give atropine I.V.

---

14. The steps in CPR outside the CCU are:

   A. _____

   <u>A</u>irway

   B. _____

   <u>B</u>reathing

   C. _____

   <u>C</u>irculation

   D. _____

   <u>D</u>efinitive therapy

15. The initial step in CPR on the general wards consists of three procedures, done almost simultaneously:

    A. _____

    B. _____

    C. _____

Vigorous blow to the precordium
Call for help

Open the airway

---

16. To open the airway and avoid obstruction by the tongue, _____ _____.

tilt the head backward

---

17. The most useful adjunct for establishing the airway is:

    A. ____ Flanged tube with bite block.

    B. ____ Oropharyngeal tube.

    C. ____ Oropharyngeal S-tube.

    D. ____ Oropharyngeal S-tube with valve.

    E. ____ Bag and mask.

A

---

18. Tracheal intubation:

    A. ____ Minimizes aspiration of gastric contents.

    B. ____ Avoids gastric distention.

    C. ____ Is easy to perform.

    D. ____ Facilitates the use of a bag for breathing.

    E. ____ Should not be attempted if it cannot be completed within 30 seconds.

A

B

D

E

19. The best way to provide ventilation during the emergency phase is _____ _____ .

mouth-to-mouth breathing

20. An endotracheal tube connected to a bag:

A. ____ Is an essential early step.

B. ____ Allows the addition of oxygen to the ventilation system.

B

C. ____ Is the best breathing adjunct after the immediate emergency.

C

21. An intermittent positive pressure breathing apparatus cannot be used during CPR unless _____ .

it is volume-cycled

22. External cardiac compression, where performed perfectly, produces a cardiac output which is ____ % of normal.

A. ____ 20%.

B. ____ 30%.

B

C. ____ 50%.

D. ____ 70%.

23. External cardiac compression when performed properly is done:

   A. _____ With the palm of the hand on the lower half of the sternum.

   B. _____ With the heel of one hand on top of the other.   *B*

   C. _____ Straddling the patient.

   D. _____ With the heel of one hand on the lower third of the sternum.   *D*

   E. _____ At the rate of 60 per minute.

   F. _____ At the rate of 60–80 per minute.   *F*

   G. _____ Displacing the sternum downward 1½ to 2 inches.   *G*

24. The best indication of the effectiveness of external cardiac compression is:

   A. _____ Pupillary size.

   B. _____ ECG.

   C. _____ Carotid artery pulsation.   *C*

   D. _____ Skin color.

   E. _____ Femoral artery pulsation.

25. The primary goal in the initial treatment of cardiac arrest is:

    A. _____ Perfusion of the coronary arteries.

    B. _____ Restoration of ventricular contraction.

    C. _____ Carotid artery pulsation.

    D. _____ Cerebral oxygenation.   *D*

---

26. External cardiac compression should never be interrupted for longer than:

    A. _____ 15 seconds.

    B. _____ 4 minutes.

    C. _____ 5 seconds.   *C*

    D. _____ 20 seconds.

---

27. The two principal advantages of a mechanical cardiopulmonary resuscitator are:

    A. _____ It is faster.

    B. _____ It frees personnel.   *B*

    C. _____ It produces a better cardiac output.   *C*

    D. _____ Resuscitation can be carried out while the patient is being moved.

    E. _____ Defibrillation can be done without interrupting resuscitation.

28. The three major types of cardiac arrest are:

  A. _____ Ventricular standstill.   A

  B. _____ Myocardial infarction.

  C. _____ Cardiovascular collapse.   C

  D. _____ Drowning.

  E. _____ Electrocution.

  F. _____ Ventricular fibrillation.   F

---

29. The most effective way to treat ventricular fibrillation initially is:

  A. _____ A 500-volt A.C. shock.

  B. _____ 100 mg. of lidocaine I.V.

  C. _____ A 400 watt-second D.C. shock.   C

  D. _____ Pronestyl® 100 mg. I.V.

---

30. Ventricular standstill may respond to:

  A. _____ Intracardiac epinephrine.   A

  B. _____ Potassium.

  C. _____ A blow to the precordium.   C

  D. _____ Quinidine.

  E. _____ A transthoracic pacing elec-   E
            trode.

  F. _____ Good myocardial oxygen-   F
            ation.

31. The first two things to do if a patient develops ventricular fibrillation and has an I.V. running are:

    A. ____ Give precordial shock with maximum voltage.

A

    B. ____ Start mouth-to-mouth breathing.

    C. ____ Give a bolus of lidocaine, 75 mg., I.V.

    D. ____ Thump the precordium.

D (A precordial thump requires only a second and occasionally reverses even ventricular fibrillation.)

---

32. Match the effects of cardiac arrest with their treatment:

    A. ____ Acidosis.

4

    B. ____ Myocardial hypotonicity and vasodilation.

1, 3, 5

    C. ____ Hypoxemia.

2, 6

    1. Epinephrine.

    2. Assisted breathing.

    3. Calcium chloride.

    4. Sodium bicarbonate.

    5. Levophed.

    6. External cardiac compression.

33. Match the arrhythmia with the drug(s) most likely to be effective in its treatment:

    A. _____ Fine ventricular fibrillation.   *4*

    B. _____ Ventricular standstill.   *3, 4*

    C. _____ Ventricular tachycardia.   *1, 5, 6*

    D. _____ Recurrent ventricular fibril-   *1, 5, 6*
             lation.

    E. _____ Sinus bradycardia.   *2*

    1. Procainamide.

    2. Atropine.

    3. Isuprel®.

    4. Epinephrine.

    5. Lidocaine.

    6. Bretylol®.

34. Resuscitation could be discontinued if:

    A. ____ The patient is over 85 years of age.

    B. ____ There is a known delay of over 10 minutes before CPR was begun.   B

    C. ____ Spontaneous respiration does not occur.   C

    D. ____ The electrocardiogram shows no electrical activity for 30 minutes.   D

    E. ____ There is no improvement of any kind in 60 minutes.   E

    F. ____ The patient has a severe fracture of the cervical spine.

35. Which three factors would help in deciding when to discontinue CPR?

    A. ____ ECG.   A

    B. ____ Deep tendon reflexes.

    C. ____ Pupillary size and reaction.   C

    D. ____ Patient's history.   D

    E. ____ EEG.

SUGGESTED READING—CHAPTER 10

1. *Emergency Measures in Cardiopulmonary Resuscitation.* American Heart Association, Committee on Cardiopulmonary Resuscitation, New York, 1969.

2. *Definitive Therapy in Cardiopulmonary Resuscitation.* American Heart Association, Committee on Cardiopulmonary Resuscitation, New York, 1971.

3. Pennington, J. E., Taylor, J. and Lown, B.: Chest thump for reverting ventricular tachycardia. *N. Eng. J. Med., 283,* 1192, 1970.

4. Lemire, J. G. and Johnson, A. L.: Is cardiac resuscitation worthwhile? A decade of experience. *N. Eng. J. Med., 286,* 970, 1972.

11

Cardioversion

Cardioversion is an elective procedure in which a brief, direct-current, precordial shock is administered at a predetermined time in the cardiac cycle.

Cardioversion is used to convert an arrhythmia to a sinus rhythm. Most commonly treated are:

1. Atrial fibrillation
2. Atrial flutter
3. Atrial tachycardia
4. Junctional (nodal) tachycardia
5. Ventricular tachycardia

It is important to recognize that some of these arrhythmias, particularly atrial tachycardia, junctional tachycardia, and ventricular tachycardia, may be due to *digitalis intoxication*. Cardioversion is generally avoided in arrhythmias due to digitalis intoxication since dangerous postshock arrhythmias may occur.

> Cardioversion is dangerous in arrhythmias due to digitalis intoxication.

Speed of action is the chief advantage of cardioversion for a dangerous arrhythmia such as ventricular tachycardia, particularly in the presence of circulatory collapse. Cardioversion is also *safer* and more likely to result in a sinus rhythm than drug therapy in other arrhythmias.

Large and possibly toxic doses of quinidine may be necessary to convert atrial fibrillation to a sinus rhythm. Large and potentially toxic doses of digitalis may be necessary to slow atrial flutter, while a small dose of current generally converts this arrhythmia to sinus rhythm.

Advantages of Cardioversion

1. Speed of action
2. Safety
3. Effectiveness

Even though electrical conversion is more likely to be effective than drug therapy, long-term success is no more likely with cardioversion than with drug conversion.

Long-term conversion is unlikely in the following clinical settings:

Long duration of atrial fibrillation
Marked cardiac or left atrial enlargement
Thyrotoxicosis
Frequently recurrent atrial tachycardia
Numerous brief bouts of arrhythmia
Intolerance for maintenance quinidine

PREPARATION FOR CARDIOVERSION

Prior to cardioversion, digitalis is discontinued for 2 to 3 days if possible. The patient is often placed on a relatively low dose of quinidine, usually 0.2 Gm. q 4 h. About 10% of patients convert to a sinus rhythm on this low dosage. Preparatory quinidine decreases the amount of current needed for conversion and the frequency of post-shock arrhythmias. This dose of quinidine is usually continued after cardioversion to help prevent reoccurrence of the initial arrhythmia.

Anesthesia or analgesia generally is used because of the discomfort associated with precordial shock. Intravenous Brevital®, Pentothal®, or Valium® are the most commonly used agents.

Steps in Elective Cardioversion

(An asterisk indicates an item which is the physician's responsibility)

* *1. Select patient.
* *2. Avoid digitalis-induced arrhythmias. Stop digitalis several days in advance.
* *3. Check serum potassium and correct hypokalemia, if present. Hypokalemia may result in post-shock arrhythmias.
* *4. Administer quinidine several days in advance. A small number of patients will convert on this drug, intolerance to the drug will be manifested, the dose of current required for conversion is reduced, and maintenance will help prevent reoccurrence of original arrhythmia.
   5. Explain the procedure to the patient.
   6. Avoid food or liquid P.O. for 6 hours prior to cardioversion.
   7. Arrange for adequate assistance for possible cardiopulmonary resuscitation (CPR). Though serious post-shock arrhythmias are uncommon, preparation for such events is always advisable in an elective procedure.
   8. Check CPR equipment.
   9. Obtain drugs which may be needed:

Epinephrine	Dilantin, injectable
Sodium bicarbonate	Digoxin, injectable
Lidocaine	Valium®, Pentothal®, or Brevital®
Quinidine	

10. Start a secure intravenous drip with a plastic intravenous catheter such as "Intracath®" or "Infusor®." The muscular contraction associated with precordial shock should not dislodge the intravenous route.

11. Apply monitoring electrodes. Select a lead axis which provides a dominant R or S wave with large amplitude. The "synchronizer" circuit will delay delivery of the precordial shock until the R wave triggers the defibrillator following closing of switch by the operator. The shock is thus *synchronized with the ECG to avoid the vulnerable period* (apex of T wave) when an electrical stimulus may produce ventricular arrhythmias such as VPC's, ventricular tachycardia, or ventricular fibrillation.

Electrodes should be located to avoid sites where the paddles will be located. Monitoring electrodes, if close to the paddles, could drain off electrical energy, causing a skin burn or failure of conversion.

12. Check equipment and synchronization. Each piece of equipment has a method to check the operation of the synchronizer.

13. Administer anesthesia.

14. Charge the defibrillator to the desired level of watt-seconds. The amount of current required is related to the type of arrhythmia. Atrial flutter often requires only low levels of current, i.e., 50 watt-seconds for conversion while atrial fibrillation may require a larger amount, 200–400 watt-seconds. The larger the current used, the more likely are post-shock arrhythmias.

15. Provide a dense field of current through the heart. This is done by avoiding dissipation of electrical energy in the skin and using adequate *paste,* proper *position* of the paddles, and firm *pressure.*

*16. Administer lidocaine or other antiarrhythmic drugs if post-shock arrhythmias occur.

17. Remain with the patient until rhythm, airway, and state of consciousness are adequate. Restart maintenance quinidine after the patient is awake.

TO PROVIDE A DENSE FIELD OF CURRENT THROUGH HEART

Paste:

Abrasive paste is better than bland cream. Apply to the paddles and rub into skin with a tongue blade. Be generous, but for reasons of electrical safety, don't smear paste on your hands and the paddle handles.

Position:

In a thin patient with prominent ribs, the need for a flat contact may dictate the location of the paddles. Generally one is to the right of the manubrium; the other is near the cardiac apex (5th left interspace, midclavicular line to posterior axillary line).

Pressure:

Firm pressure flattens out skin folds and insures that the entire paddle surface (not just an edge) is in contact with the skin.

ILLUSTRATIVE CASES

Precordial Shock in the Treatment of Arrhythmias Complicating Myocardial Infarction

1. A 48-year-old man with acute infarction remained quite ill during his first 3 days in the CCU. Temperature was 102°, blood pressure 105/70, PCWP stable at about 12 mm.Hg., and urine volume adequate. He preferred to have the head of the bed elevated but had no definite signs of heart failure. He had received no digitalis. Lead II on admission indicated a sinus rhythm with a rate of 82.

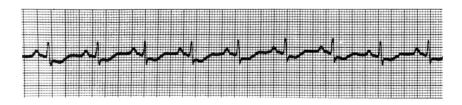

At 6:00 A.M. on the 4th day, his heart rate suddenly rose to 148. He felt no worse, though the blood pressure fell slightly. This was the monitoring lead rhythm strip:

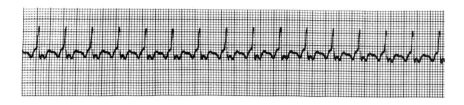

(1) Identify the errors in the nurse's ECG description.

Technique satisfactory.	*Correct.*
Ventricular rate 150/min.	*Correct.*
Ventricular rhythm regular.	*Correct.*
QRS duration 0.08 sec.	*Correct.*
Atrial rate 150/min.	*Wrong. The rate is 300.*
Atrial rhythm regular.	*Correct.*
PR interval 0.14 sec.	*Correct, in part.*
A-V conduction normal. Each P is followed by a QRS, the PR interval is normal and constant.	*Wrong. Every other P wave is not conducted.*

The doctor's first request was: "Measure the interval between the suspected atrial waves. Now divide this interval in half. Could there be another deflection halfway between the obvious ones?"

(2) Interval between obvious atrial waves.	*0.40 sec.*
Divide by two.	*0.20 sec.*
Could there be another deflection between the obvious ones?	*Yes*
(3) What is the arrhythmia?	*Atrial flutter with 2:1 block.*

The next question was: "Has he had anything to eat since bedtime?" The answer was "No," and the nurse was asked to get things ready for cardioversion.

(4) List some of the nursing responsibilities to be accomplished during the 15-minute period while waiting for the physician to arrive.

_____ *Explain coming events.*

_____ *Check security of the I.V. drip.*

_____ *Request the presence of an*

_____ *additional person.*

_____ *Assemble drugs and supplies*

_____ *at bedside.*

The doctor assisted her with cardioversion about 35 minutes after the tachycardia arose.

(5) What might have influenced the physician to proceed with cardioversion instead of rapid digitalization?

_____

_____

_____

_____

Cardioversion ordinarily will terminate atrial flutter promptly and safely. Giving fractional doses of an I.V. digitalis preparation may require hours of careful bedside observation. If digitalis toxicity should arise before the ventricular rate is slowed, then there is a real problem. Cardioversion at that point may be risky.

(6) Why didn't the doctor give a phone order for stat cardioversion by the nurse?

_____

_____

Arrhythmia was not immediately life-threatening. The patient needed anesthesia. The physician wanted to confirm ECG diagnosis.

(7) What complications would you expect in this patient if the ventricular rate remained 150 for several hours?

Congestive failure and shock.

(8) Why?

During tachycardia, diastole is short. Ventricular filling and coronary blood flow both occur during diastole. Cardiac output suffers.

2. A 62-year-old man with aortic stenosis and a fresh infarction appeared to be in good condition until he became stuporous, cold, and clammy within a few minutes after developing this arrhythmia. The blood pressure could not be measured but a faint femoral pulse sometimes was palpable.

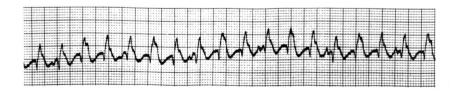

(1) Summarize the nurse's ECG description.

"We have a regular ventricular rhythm at a rate of about 165. The QRS is broad. This is a ventricular tachycardia or . . ." The doctor interrupted somewhat curtly.

(2) Why?

_____

_____

The patient was failing rapidly. This was not the time for an erudite discussion of ventricular tachycardia vs. supraventricular tachycardia with bundle branch block.
He ordered an I.V. push dose of 100 mg. lidocaine, to be followed in two minutes by cardioversion if tachycardia persisted, another physician were not at the bedside and the patient remained stuporous, cold, and pulseless.

(3) Why did he wish the nurse to proceed within a very few minutes?

_____

_____

In this patient, tachycardia producing vascular collapse probably will be fatal quite soon.

SUGGESTED READING—CHAPTER 11

1. Resnekov, L.: Present status of electroversion in the management of cardiac dysrhythmias. *Circulation, 47,* 1356, 1973.

2. Lown, B.: Electrical reversion of cardiac arrhythmias. *Br. Heart J., 29,* 469, 1967.

3. Rossi, M. and Lown, B.: The use of quinidine in cardioversion. *Amer. J. Cardiol., 19,* 234, 1967.

4. Sussman, R. M., *et al.*: Myocardial changes after direct-current electroshock. *J. Amer. Med. Assn., 189,* 739, 1964.

12

Pacing and pacemakers

PACEMAKER

Electrodes

An electrode is an electrical conductor which makes contact between the body and the recording or stimulating apparatus. An electrode may be either *external*—on the surface of the body, or *internal*.

Internal electrodes are of two types: *Epicardial,* on the surface of the heart, and *endocardial,* inside a cardiac chamber, usually the right ventricle. *Endocardial* electrodes are placed within the cardiac chamber by two means, *transvenous catheter* and *percutaneous transventricular puncture.*

Transvenous catheter method: A flexible tube (similar to a urethral catheter) is advanced through a vein until the electrode(s) at the tip contact the inner lining of the atrium or ventricle.

1. *Unipolar electrode catheter:* Only one wire in the catheter and one electrode at the tip. The *indifferent electrode* is placed anywhere on the body surface.
2. *Bipolar electrode catheter:* Two wires and two electrodes, contained in one covering.

Percutaneous transventricular method. A needle containing a wire is advanced through the skin into the heart chamber. The needle is then removed, leaving the wire impinged upon the endocardium.

Positive and negative poles: Labeled connections of the pulse generator. Usually the negative pole of the pulse generator is connected to the unipolar catheter, and the positive pole to the indifferent electrode. A *bipolar catheter* may be connected with either electrode to either pole. Usually the negative pole to the tip of the catheter results in a lower threshold.

Pulse Generator

A *pulse generator* is an electrical device which periodically releases a brief burst of electrical current (a "pulse"). When conducted to the heart, this electrical "pulse" may produce a heart beat. A pulse generator may be either *external*—outside the body, or *internal*—implanted in a subcutaneous pocket.

The *amplitude control* furnishes an adjustment to vary the strength of the stimulating current, sometimes expressed as volts, amperes, or joules. The *rate control* allows adjustment of the heart rate.

Miscellaneous Terms

Overdrive: Use of pacemaking at a rate above the intrinsic rate to suppress an ectopic focus.

Demand mode: Circuitry which causes the pulse generator to release a stimulus only if the interval between the spontaneous QRS complexes exceeds a pre-set limit. The pulse generator fires if the demand arises (heart rate slow) but does not fire if a spontaneous beat occurs.

Standby mode: Circuitry which turns on the pulse generator if the heart rate drops below the preset limits. The generator will continue to operate until turned off.

Threshold current: The strength of pacing current needed to initiate a depolarization wave.

Pacer blip: An electrocardiographic deflection produced by the pacing current. The pacing blip will be followed by a depolarization wave (QRS complex) if the stimulus exceeds the threshold level for that particular moment of the cardiac cycle (see *refractory period* below).

Capture: Each pacing stimulus produces a depolarization wave. "Noncapture" may be due to a stimulus of subthreshold strength, or to a stimulus occurring during the refractory period.

Competition: Some of the depolarization waves are initiated by the pacing stimuli, others by the intrinsic cardiac pacemaker.

Refractory period: A portion of the cardiac cycle during which a stimulus will not result in a depolarization wave. Actually, the *threshold* varies throughout the cardiac cycle. The threshold is high from the onset of QRS to the onset of the T wave; a pacer blip occurring during this phase usually will not result in capture. The threshold is lower during the diastolic period between T and the following QRS. The threshold is abnormally low during the *supernormal refractory or "vulnerable" period,* usually coinciding with the apex of the T wave. The heart is vulnerable to ventricular fibrillation if a stimulus of sufficient strength and duration is delivered during the *supernormal refractory period.*

Line-powered: An electrical device which receives its power from the electrical lines in the building.

Battery-powered: An electrical device which receives its power from a battery.

INTERNAL PACEMAKING

Internal pacing may be provided by *epicardial electrodes* sutured to the surface of the heart which has been exposed by thoracotomy. This is not suitable for the patient with recent myocardial infarction but rather is a method of managing complete heart block in patients able to tolerate a small thoracotomy.

Transvenous internal pacing is the method of choice in the CCU. Because of little discomfort, disturbance, or risk to the patient, a transvenous pacing catheter often is inserted at the earliest suspicion that it may be needed.

Several types of transvenous catheters are available. A *unipolar transvenous pacing catheter* may be introduced via a plastic needle in the basilic, subclavian, or femoral vein. A venous cutdown may be needed. The catheter may be guided into the right ventricle, using the ECG pattern recorded from its tip to guide its placement. A unipolar catheter contains one wire which delivers the stimulating currents from the pulse generator to the lining of the right ventricle (endocardium). A second wire (indifferent electrode) is sutured to the skin and serves to complete the circuit between the heart and the pulse generator.

Most commonly a *bipolar transvenous pacing catheter,* containing two wires, is used. It may be introduced through a needle, but often a venous cutdown is needed. Fluoroscopy can be used to guide it into the right ventricle but placement using the ECG pattern also can be done. A chest x-ray should be obtained following placement.

The *percutaneous, transventricular* internal pacing technique is useful in an emergency. A long needle is prepared with a thin stainless steel wire protruding ¼ inch through the tip and bent over, as a fishhook. The needle and its wire are inserted through the skin overlying the heart and advanced into the chamber of the right or left ventricle. The needle is withdrawn, leaving the bentover tip of the wire impinged on the endocardium. This wire and an indifferent electrode to complete the circuit are then connected to the pulse generator. The whole procedure requires only a few moments and can be done with less risk than that offered by untreated heart block. This emergency procedure allows treatment of heart block or ventricular standstill until a transvenous pacing catheter can be introduced. When the emergency wire is no longer needed, it can be withdrawn with a gentle tug. Such pacing catheters are commercially available.

Indications for Insertion of a Pacing Catheter

A pacing catheter may be introduced to:

1. Obtain an intracavitary ECG.
2. Treat A-V block.
3. Drive the heart at a faster rate to suppress an ectopic focus.

Intracavitary ECG: Identification of P waves is crucial for the diagnosis of many arrhythmias, and rational treatment requires accurate diagnosis. Ventricular tachycardia, for instance, ordinarily will be treated with precordial shock; atrial tachycardia or flutter may need quite a different approach. Electrocardiographic features may be similar until P waves are identified (A-V dissociation is a common feature of ventricular tachycardia).

When tachycardia is present, P waves may be hidden by the larger QRS complexes and T waves recorded in any of the 12 standard levels. A recording from the electrode tip of a pacing catheter within the right atrium will show P waves large enough to identify.

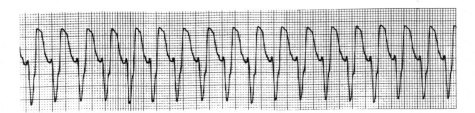

Monitoring lead. A regular tachycardia is present. Is this ventricular tachycardia, supraventricular tachycardia with aberrant ventricular conduction, or atrial flutter with 2:1 block and aberrant ventricular conduction?

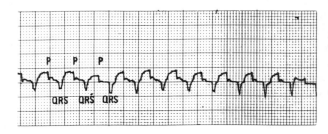

Intracavitary lead, recorded from the right atrium. A-V dissociation is not present. P waves bear a constant relationship to the QRS complexes. Probably this is a supraventricular tachycardia.

A-V Block: This is the most common indication for insertion of a pacing catheter. The influence on cardiac dynamics, prognosis, and need for pacing is somewhat determined by the site of coronary artery occlusion and myocardial infarction.

The A-V node receives its blood supply from the right coronary artery in about 90% of individuals. When A-V block occurs with right coronary artery occlusion and *inferior myocardial infarction,* the block is probably due to *A-V nodal ischemia.* The amount of tissue damage is small, the duration of block brief, and prognosis good. A-V block associated with left-anterior-descending-artery occlusion and *anterior myocardial infarction* probably is due to *necrosis* of the bundle branches. The associated infarction is large, duration of block prolonged, and prognosis poor.

A pacing catheter usually is inserted for third degree A-V block with either inferior (posterior) or anterior infarctions and may be summarized as follows:

Characteristics	Inferior Myocardial Infarction	Anterior Myocardial Infarction
Site of block	A-V node	Bundle branches
Process	Ischemic	Necrotic
Onset	Gradual	Sudden
If second degree block	Mobitz Type I (Wenckebach)	Mobitz Type II
If third degree block		
a. Pacemaker	A-V junction	Idioventricular
b. QRS complex	Narrow, normal	Wide, bizarre
c. Rate	40–55/min.	25–35/min.
d. Stability of		
escape focus	Stable	Unstable
Duration	Temporary	Permanent
Prognosis	Poor	Very poor
Pacemaker insertion	Sometimes	Usually
Adams-Stokes attacks	Rare	Common

A *standby pacing catheter* usually is indicated if infarction is complicated by:

1. First degree A-V block with bundle branch block.
2. Second degree A-V block of Mobitz Type II.
3. Right bundle branch block with left anterior (superior) hemiblock or left posterior (inferior) hemiblock.
4. New right bundle branch block in anterior infarction.
5. New left bundle branch block.
6. Sinus bradycardia or slow junctional rhythm with clinical signs of hypoperfusion.

Observation and drug therapy with atropine is usually indicated in:

1. First degree A-V block with normal intraventricular conduction.
2. Second degree A-V block of Mobitz Type I (Wenckebach).
3. Old right or left bundle branch block without other conduction disorder.

"Overdrive" treatment of arrhythmias: Even though the ventricular rate seems reasonable, it may be inadequate to suppress ectopic foci. If a faster-than-normal rate is produced by pacing, ectopic tachycardias or recurrent ventricular fibrillation may be prevented.

Testing Pacemaker Threshold

Purpose: To determine how much current is required to stimulate the ventricle. It is important to know that the pacemaker will indeed function satisfactorily, should the need arise. If the threshold is high (above 4 to 6 ma), probably the catheter tip is not positioned properly within the right ventricle. If pacing cannot be accomplished, the catheter tip may have moved back into the atrium or may have passed into the pulmonary artery. The pacemaker threshold should be checked daily.

Technique: Observe the patient carefully during the procedure. Be prepared to proceed rapidly in providing an adequate pacemaking stimulus. *If the patient is dependent upon the pacemaker,* start by running a brief ECG strip, noting the current strength. Then reduce the strength stepwise, one ma at a time, running a brief strip at each strength. Soon you will reach a current amplitude which is inadequate to stimulate. The "threshold" is the lowest current which results in a paced QRS complex for each pacer impulse.

If the patient is not dependent upon the pacemaker, set the pacemaker rate control at a rate slightly faster than the patient's own rate, set the current amplitude to zero, and turn the pacer on. Advance the current strength stepwise in one ma increments until each pacer blip is followed by a paced QRS complex. The lowest amount of current which captures the ventricular rhythm is the "threshold."

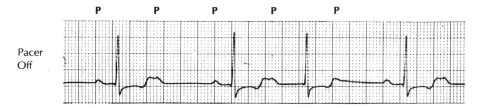

Pacer
Off

The atrial rate is 88. The first P wave is conducted with a PR interval of 0.22 sec. The second P wave is partially hidden on the downslope of the first T wave. The third P wave is conducted, with a PR of 0.20 sec. The fourth P wave also is conducted, with a PR of 0.40 sec. The fifth P wave is hidden in the T of the third QRS cycle and is not conducted. The sixth P wave is conducted, with a PR of 0.22 sec. This is an example of second degree A-V heart block and illustrates the Wenckebach phenomenon.

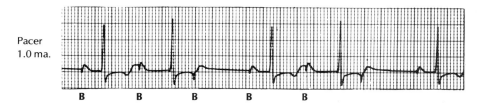

Pacer
1.0 ma.

The pacemaker has been turned on. Note the pacer blips at a rate of 90. The current strength is 1.0 ma. There is no capture.

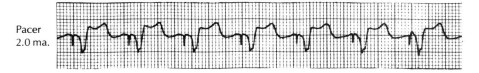

Pacer
2.0 ma.

The pacing stimulus has been increased to 2.0 ma. Each pacer blip is followed by a QRS complex. Because the QRS complexes arise from an ectopic focus (the pacing electrode), they are broad and quite different from those which result from an impulse reaching the ventricles via the normal conduction pathways. The threshold is 2.0 ma.

PACING TECHNIQUES

General Term	Electrodes	Techniques of Positioning	Pulse Generator	Problems and Comments	Use in Acute Myocardial Infarction
Epicardial pacing	Two wires sutured into surface of ventricle.	Thoracotomy.	Buried in subcutaneous pocket. "Demand" or fixed.	Thoracotomy needed. Method for chronic complete A-V block in good risk patient. Pulse generator replacement required after 12–36 months.	None. Complete block following M.I. seldom is permanent.
Endocardial pacing	Bipolar or unipolar pacing catheter.	Via vein, into right ventricle. Guidance from fluoroscopy, or from ECG pattern recorded from tip of catheter.	Battery-operated safest. "Demand" or fixed. External or implanted.	Fluoroscopic guidance: transportation of sick patient to X-ray Dept. ECG guidance: 15–35% failure. Transvenous endocardial electrode with implanted pulse generator is usual "permanent" method for chronic, complete A-V block.	Common. Little hazard. Usually inserted *before* serious degree of A-V block develops.
Percutaneous transventricular pacing	Wire, insulated or bare.	Wire placed in ventricle via needle introduced through chest wall.	External. Battery operated safest.	Rapid. No special equipment or skill needed. Danger of bleeding or coronary artery damage less than danger of poorly managed A-V block.	Emergency, or if no facilities for transvenous catheter introduction.

Pacing Malfunction

Failure of temporary transvenous pacing is usually due to poor position of the electrode at the myocardium or a change in myocardial threshold. In both instances pacing is usually intermittent and the pacing stimulus is present. Increasing the output of the pulse generator may lead to adequate pacing. Temporary help may be obtained by keeping the patient in a particular position where capture is improved. Repositioning of the catheter generally is necessary.

In pacing failure with a pacing stimulus present:

1. Increase pulse generator output.
2. Try to obtain capture by moving the patient into a different position.
3. Reposition the pacing catheter.

Occasionally pacemaker failure may be due to pulse generator malfunction or a defect, such as wire breakage or a short circuit in the pacing catheter. In both instances a pacing stimulus is absent, at least intermittently.

Competency of the pacing catheter may be tested by recording an endocardial electrocardiogram from each pole in a bipolar catheter, attaching the V lead to each pole in sequence and a bipolar electrocardiogram from both poles by connecting to Lead I of the electrocardiograph.

In pacing failure with a pacing stimulus absent:

1. Check for failure of the pulse generator.
2. Check for a defect in the pacing catheter.

QUESTIONS—CHAPTER 12

1. In the coronary care unit, internal pacing is usually done using a _____ electrode.

   transvenous endocardial

2. A unipolar catheter contains an electrode at the tip and a single wire. To complete the circuit, what is required?

   _____

   _____

   _____

   _____

   An indifferent electrode, usually attached to the skin of the chest or arm.

3. The purpose of a pulse generator is to:

   ____ A. Improve the pulse when it is weak.

   ____ B. Produce small voltage shocks.

   ____ C. Provide emergency lighting in the event of a power failure.

   B

4. Pacing may be used for:

   A. _____

   Ventricular standstill.

   B. _____

   Low ventricular rate due to A-V block.

   C. _____

   Suppression of an ectopic rhythm.

5. Adams-Stokes attacks occur because of

    _____

    _____

    _____ .

    cerebral ischemia due to low cardiac output

    They are usually associated with a (slow) (fast) rate.

    slow

6. A transvenous pacing catheter may be used for:

    A. _____

    Endocardial ECG to identify P waves

    B. _____

    Treatment of A-V block

    C. _____

    Suppression of ectopic focus by overdrive

7. Overdrive means:

    ____ A. A high gear ratio in an automobile transmission.

    ____ B. Suppression of an ectopic focus by pacing the heart at a faster rate.

    B

    ____ C. Treatment of 2:1 A-V block by internal pacing.

8. Transvenous pacing is tolerated well by the patient and is highly effective. Disadvantages include:

A. _____

The electrode must be inserted in advance

B. _____

The electrode must be protected from stray currents (See Chapter 13)

9. What arrhythmias commonly occur when the catheter tip enters the ventricle?_____

_____

_____

_____

Ventricular premature beats, ventricular tachycardia, ventricular fibrillation.

10. A 56-year-old male is admitted with an acute inferior myocardial infarction. The PR interval is initially 0.18 seconds. When the PR interval increases to 0.24 seconds, a transvenous catheter is introduced. As the catheter enters the right ventricle, this ECG pattern is observed:

What is the arrhythmia?

_____

Ventricular fibrillation.

What is the treatment?

_____

Precordial shock.

What should be ruled out before further manipulation of the catheter is done?

_____

_____

_____

Rule out the presence of stray electrical current. (See Chapter 13.)

---

11. If the patient is dependent on the pacemaker, the threshold should be determined by:

_____ A. Reducing the amplitude gradually till capture is lost.

_____ B. Gradually slowing the rate till pacing no longer occurs.

_____ C. Increasing the amplitude from zero in increments till each pacer blip is followed by a QRS.

A

SUGGESTED READING—CHAPTER 12

1. Del Negro, A. A. and Fletcher, R. D.: Indications for and use of artificial cardiac pacemakers: Part II. *Current Problems in Cardiology III,* No. 8. Year Book Medical Publishers, Chicago, 1978.

2. Chatterjee, K., Swan, H. J. C., Ganz, W., Gray, R., Loebel, H., Forrester, J. S. and Chonette, D.: Use of a balloon-tipped flotation electrode catheter for cardiac monitoring. *Amer. J. Cardiol., 36,* 56, 1975.

3. Ritter, W. S., Atkins, J. M., Blomquist, C. G. and Mullins, C. B.: Permanent pacing in patients with transient trifascicular block during myocardial infarction. *Amer. J. Cardiol., 38,* 205, 1976.

4. Waugh, R. A., Wagner, G. S., Hanley, T. L., *et al.:* Immediate and remote prognostic significance of fascicular block during acute myocardial infarction. *Circulation, 47,* 765, 1973.

5. Resnekov, L. and Lipp, H.: Pacemaking and acute myocardial infarction. *Prog. Cardiovasc. Dis., 14,* 475, 1972.

6. Hamilton, A. J.: *Selected Subjects for Critical Care Nurses,* Chapter 5, page 114, Pacemakers. Mountain Press Publishing Co., Missoula, Mt., 1975.

13

Electrical safety

PRINCIPLES OF ELECTRICITY

Electric *current* consists of electrons flowing through a conductor, such as a wire or a salty solution. All conductors have some opposition to the flow of current; this opposition is known as *resistance*. *Voltage* may be thought of as the push which tends to move current through a conductor, despite its resistance.

These concepts can be illustrated by the flow of water *(current)* through a pipe *(resistance)* leading from a reservoir with a standing head of pressure *(voltage)*.

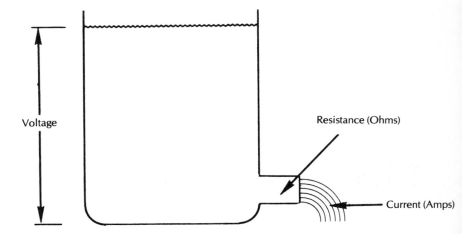

The German physicist, G. S. Ohm, described the relationship between voltage, resistance, and current. Current is the feature responsible for electrical hazards to the heart. Therefore we express Ohm's Law in the following fashion:

Ohm's Law: Current $= \dfrac{\text{Voltage}}{\text{Resistance}}$ $\qquad I = \dfrac{E}{R}$

Examination of the equation shows that if the resistance is large, current will be low, even with a fairly high voltage. Conversely, even with a low voltage, current can be large if the resistance is very low.

An Explanation of Electrical Terms

A.C. (Alternating Current): An electrical current which periodically reverses its direction of flow. In the United States, alternating current reverses its direction 60 times a second.

D.C. (Direct Current): An electrical current flowing in one direction continuously.

Watt: An electrical measure of "power," analogous to "horsepower."

Ampere: A measure of electrical flow or current. One ampere is equal to 1000 milliamperes or 1,000,000 microamperes.

Ohm: A measure of resistance to electrical flow.

Volt: A measure of electrical force.

Charge: Electrical particles which are stored up and not flowing, as in a flashlight battery. This is analogous to water stored behind a dam.

Capacitor: An electrical device which allows the storage of an electrical charge, often with high power and voltage.

Stray Current: Current which has leaked from its usual pathway in a piece of electrical equipment and is flowing through other parts, such as the chassis. This current is not being used to operate the equipment and may actually interfere with its function. Stray current is responsible for the "shock" you get when you handle an electrical instrument which is faulty.

Ground: A connection of an electrical circuit or piece of equipment with the earth. A ground is designed to drain stray current away from an electrical instrument. In modern instruments, this is done by providing a power cable with three wires. The third wire is the ground. It is connected to the eccentric prong on the power plug. If a "cheater" or adapter is used, proper grounding is prevented.

Current Density: The amount of current which passes through a certain area.

Murphy's Law: If anything can go wrong, it will.

SAFETY FACTORS

$$\text{Current} = \frac{\text{Voltage}}{\text{Resistance}}$$

Even substantial voltage applied to the *surface* of the body generally does not cause fatal arrhythmia. Two safety factors protect us somewhat when voltage is applied to the *surface* of the body:

1. *Dry skin provides a large resistance.*

   A shock from your percolator will cause pain, fright, muscle contraction, and perhaps a burn; but it is not likely to be fatal. Although you receive 120 volts, the 100,000 ohm skin resistance indicates a current flow of only 0.00120 amperes.

2. *Low current density.*

   More important, when current flows between two surface points (your hand on the percolator and your foot on the floor connected to the earth), current which gets into the body spreads diffusely, forming a large number of lines of force. The number of these lines at a given point describes the "current density." The density is high at the point of application of the current. In Figure 1 (next page), note the low current density at the heart when current flows from one point on the body surface to another point on the body surface.

ELECTRICAL SAFETY WITH LOW VOLTAGE

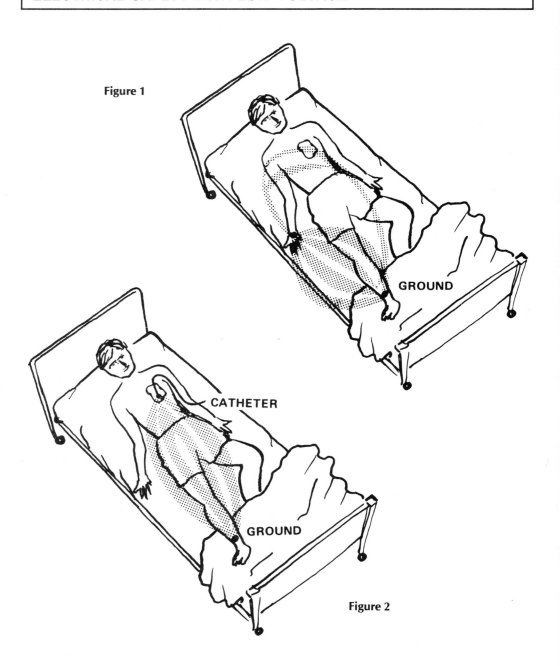

Figure 1

CATHETER

GROUND

GROUND

Figure 2

Two common procedures in coronary care circumvent these protective characteristics. These coronary care procedures permit:

1. Bypassing skin resistance.
2. High current density in the heart.
    A. Transvenous pacing. The tip of the pacing catheter is in contact with the right ventricle. Any voltage applied to the exterior terminal of the pacing wire finds extremely low resistance; thus a large current can flow. Furthermore, the tip of the pacing wire provides an extremely high current density at that small point (Figure 2). Even 20 millionths of an ampere applied directly to the heart may cause ventricular fibrillation. The flow is from the pacing-catheter electrode through the heart muscle and out the ground wire of the monitoring equipment to the earth.
    B. Intracardiac electrocardiography. An electrocardiogram may be recorded from inside the heart in order to better understand an arrhythmia. An electrode wire is introduced into the heart chambers through a peripheral vein. Again, a conductor with low resistance bypasses the usual protective insulation at the body surface; and the current density is high at the tip of a recording electrode.

Ventricular fibrillation may be produced by minute amounts of electrical current when applied directly to the myocardium.

Most line-operated equipment has some stray current on the chassis. Even the nurse at the bedside may be a source of alternating current, picking up electrical waves passing through the air just as an antenna picks up radio waves.

If this stray current is applied to the end of the pacing catheter in the ventricle, ventricular fibrillation may result if the current can flow from the catheter tip to the earth. Even if the patient is not connected to the ground via a normally-applied electrode, one must assume that he may be grounded through numerous channels—the bed frame, damp sheets touching the bed frame and the floor, another person at the bedside connecting the patient to a grounded radiator, oxygen line, or suction machine.

Furthermore, current may flow from any piece of electrical apparatus connected to the patient from the body surface through the heart to the pacing catheter electrode. Lethal current will flow if the catheter then permits an escape route to ground, such as touching a bedrail or a doctor's hand.

Particular danger arises when two items of electrical equipment, such as an ECG machine and a suction machine, are attached simultaneously to a patient with a transvenous pacing catheter. If improperly grounded, current may flow from one machine to the other by way of the pacing catheter.

> When a patient with a transvenous or transthoracic pacing catheter develops ventricular fibrillation, the arrhythmia should be attributed to stray current until proven otherwise.

ELECTRICAL SAFETY IN THE CCU

Despite the complexity of electricity, principles of electrical safety are very simple.

Checklist for Electrical Safety in the CCU

1. Recognize that the average electrician is thinking in terms of *macroshock* when he checks to see that the electrical system is safe. You must be thinking of *microshock*.

2. An electrician trained in the fundamentals of microshock safety should check all electrical equipment in the CCU at regular intervals. Wire insulation, plugs, and the grounding terminal will receive particular scrutiny.

3. Check for stray current in all electrical equipment brought into the CCU.

4. Ensure that the same potential is present at the ground wire of all objects in the patient's environment. An "equipotential bus" is simply a high-quality ground connecting all surfaces with which the patient or anyone who touches the patient are grounded and will be at the same potential.

5. Permit no electric beds in the CCU.

6. Permit no equipment without a three-pronged plug.

7. Outlaw adapters for three-prong plugs. Never let in a cheater.

8. Protect exposed terminals of pacing catheters from stray current. Insertion into a rubber glove is an easy method.

9. Use rubber gloves to handle the exposed terminal of the pacing catheter.

10. Avoid use of more than one piece of line-powered equipment when a pacing catheter is in place. If several items are essential, each must be connected to a common ground.

11. Recognize that sixty-cycle interference on the monitor or ECG may indicate stray current.
12. Pace with a battery-operated device unless you are sure that a line-operated pacemaker is isolated from ground.
13. If ventricular fibrillation occurs during cardiac pacing or pacing catheter insertion, consider that it is due to stray current until proven otherwise.

Electrical Safety with High Voltage

High voltage as used in precordial shock has hazards both to the patient and to the personnel in the CCU.

Precordial shock, improperly administered, may produce severe skin burns.

To avoid skin burns:

1. Use adequate "gritty" electrode paste or saline-soaked pads. Avoid creams.
2. Apply the paddles firmly and flatly against the chest. Avoid gentle application or application with only the edge of the paddle against the skin.
3. Don't place paddles too close to the ground electrode of the monitoring system. Considerable electrical energy may pass through the smaller electrode, causing a burn or draining off so much electrical energy that the treatment is ineffective.

Measures should be taken to avoid accidental shock of the staff.

To avoid accidental shock:

1. Once the defibrillator is charged, caution should be used to avoid accidental discharge.
2. When the precordial shock is administered, be careful that no one is in contact with the patient or bed.

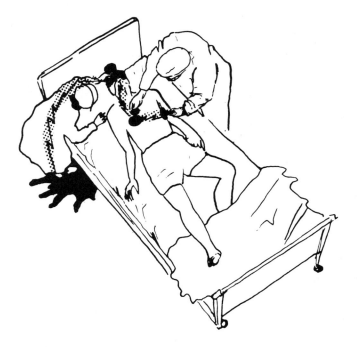

Current will flow to the rescuer if the rescuer's body is grounded (as touching a grounded bed or foot in saline or urine and there is contact with the patient).

QUESTIONS—CHAPTER 13

1. Ohm's law states:

   A. ____ Current equals voltage times resistance.

   B. ____ Resistance equals voltage times current.

   C. ____ $Current = \dfrac{Voltage}{Resistance}$

   C

2. Examination of this equation reveals that if the resistance is large, the current will be:

   A. ____ Large.

   B. ____ Small.

   B

3. Even though voltage is very low, current could be large if resistance is _____.

   low.

4. Stray current is current which _____ _____ _____ _____

   has leaked from its usual pathway and is flowing to other parts of the equipment.

   Stray current can be eliminated with:

   A. ____ A voltmeter.

   B. ____ Transvenous pacing.

   C. ____ Proper grounding.

   C

5. Two modern techniques which bypass the protective resistance normally provided by the skin and subcutaneous tissue are:

    A. _____   *Transvenous pacing*

    B. _____   *Intracardiac electrocardiography*

6. Small amounts of electrical current applied to the myocardium may result in _____   *ventricular fibrillation.*

    _____.

7. The leakage of current from faulty equipment may result in ventricular fibrillation during:

    A. ____ Precordial shock.

    B. ____ Transvenous pacing.   *B*

    C. ____ Lidocaine infusion.

8. A patient is connected to an ECG and a suction machine. Now a pacing catheter is advanced from an arm vein to the heart. Stray current could reach the heart through _____.   *the pacing catheter.*

9. Ventricular fibrillation occurring in a patient receiving cardiac pacing should be considered due to _____.   *leakage of stray current.*

10.

The artifact on the above ECG is due to
_____ .

60 cycle current.

It means:

A. _____ .

Stray current is present.

B. _____ .

Grounding is inadequate.

---

11. Proper grounding is accomplished by:

A. _____

_____ .

Proper grounding of electrical circuits by the electrician.

B. _____

_____ .

Use of three-prong plugs.

---

12. All electrical equipment in the coronary care unit should be checked periodically with a _____ .

voltmeter.

---

13. The exposed terminals of a pacing catheter should be protected from stray current by:

A. ____ Wearing rubber gloves when handling.

A

B. ____ Insertion of the ends in a rubber glove.

B

C. ____ Covering the site of insertion with a dry dressing.

14. Skin burns from precordial shock may be avoided by:

   A. _____
      _____ .

   Use of "gritty" electrode paste on the paddles and skin.

   B. _____
      _____ .

   Application of the paddles firmly and flatly against the chest.

   C. _____
      _____ .

   Avoiding placement of paddles close to monitoring electrodes.

15. Accidental shock of the staff can be avoided by:

   A. _____
      _____ .

   Using caution once the defibrillator is charged.

   B. _____
      _____ .

   Avoiding contact with the patient when precordial shock is administered.

SUGGESTED READING—CHAPTER 13

1. Arbeit, S. R., Parker, B. and Rubin, I. L.: Controlling the electrocution hazard in the hospital. *J. Amer. Med. Assn., 220,* 1581, 1972.

2. Kilpatrick, D. G.: The electrical environment. *The Med. Clin. No. Amer., 55,* 1095, 1971.

3. Merkel, R. and Sovie, M. D.: Electrocution hazards with transvenous pacemaker electrodes. *Amer. J. Nursing, 68,* 2560, 1968.

4. Starmer, C. F., Whalen, R. E. and McIntosh, H. D.: Hazards of electric shock in cardiology. *Amer. J. Cardiol., 14,* 537, 1964.

5. Whalen, R. E. and Starmer, C. F.: Electric shock hazards in clinical cardiology. *Mod. Concepts Cardiovasc. Dis., 36,* 7, 1967.

14

The patient's reaction to his illness

Throughout history, the heart has been a symbol of physical strength and integrity. Its role as a "vital" organ is entrenched in our culture.

ANXIETY

A myocardial infarction is a major emotional problem in every patient. Its frequency as a cause of disability and death causes *fear*. Different individuals react differently to similar circumstances. Sex, age, social status, background, and personal experiences all may modify emotional reactions. But in all, a heart attack causes fear and is a threat of death, unemployment, and restricted activity, to mention a few effects.

Threats and fear produce anxiety.

Anxiety causes increased heart rate, blood pressure, myocardial oxygen consumption, and myocardial work. Circulating epinephrine and norepinephrine are heightened. During anxiety, a higher incidence of arrhythmias have been noted, possibly related to enhanced levels of these circulating sympathetic hormones or the increase in myocardial work.

Early experiences with patients in intensive care units, recovery rooms and coronary care units demonstrated a high incidence of *restlessness, agitation, insomnia, fantasies, hallucinations, and delirium.* These symptoms are related to anxiety, fear, preoccupation with death, lack of sleep, a strange environment, and excessive sedation.

Much of the patient's anxiety and fear can be relieved by adequate explanation of his situation to him and his family, frequent reassurance, a supportive atmosphere, and discussion of concerns which the patient is encouraged to volunteer. *Talking with the patient about his anxieties immediately reduces their threat.* Explanation should be optimistic and reassuring but sincere, mature, and truthful.

HOSTILITY, ANGER, AND DENIAL

The acute phase of myocardial infarction produces major disturbances in the patient's relation with others. Imagine the situation of the usually self-sufficient, aggressive, dynamic individual who suddenly must passively submit to being undressed, dressed, washed, fed, turned, and helped with toilet activities. Under orders, he is subjected to a regimen that could only be termed as "being treated like a baby." Such a patient is likely to react with hostility and anger or will deny the significance of the illness.

Hostility, anger, and denial of illness often are followed by depression.

Many patients have a depressive reaction in the weeks following a myocardial infarction. Optimistic reassurance and a supportive atmosphere can reduce the severity of depression and lead to earlier rehabilitation of the patient.

THE FAMILY

Most coronary care units allow visiting for short periods and limit visits to the family. Family members are anxious, confused, and frightened; sometimes they are even afraid to touch their loved one. The wife sees her husband wired to a strange box where wiggly lines glow across the screen. An intravenous solution is connected to his arm, an oxygen mask covers his face. She can't even sit down for there is no room for a chair. The amazing thing is how well the family usually does in this type of situation. An understanding, compassionate nurse who can give a reassuring explanation of the coronary care unit and the patient's illness is indeed an angel in white.

REHABILITATION

Rehabilitation is often thought of as something that begins during the convalescent stage of a myocardial infarction. In fact, rehabilitation should begin as soon as the patient reaches medical care. Again, the proper attitude for the physician and the nurse are of paramount importance. Almost every patient with a postcoronary rehabilitation problem has a major emotional disturbance; often inappropriate remarks of some member of the medical team have been a contributing factor.

The patient with myocardial infarction can be helped to understand his problem if his illness is compared with a fractured femur. There is pain initially, but not all pain represents further damage. A period of rest is necessary for satisfactory healing of the local injury in both instances.

Finally, rehabilitation includes a period of gradually increasing physical activity to return the injured organ to its full function.

Rehabilitation includes participation of the family. If the family understands the diagnosis, prognosis, nature of healing, and the rehabilitation program, overconcern and overprotection are avoided. A smoother return to useful activity by the patient will be the result.

The patient with uncomplicated "average" myocardial infarction will have little pain after the first 24 hours. He may feed himself and probably use a bedside commode which is less strenuous for him than a bedpan. After three to five days, many patients can be transferred to less intensive care.

Significant arrhythmias may occur in the convalescent period. Many hospitals continue to monitor the patient's cardiac rhythm following transfer from the coronary care unit, employing small portable monitors which transmit the electrocardiogram by telemetry to a central station. After the first week, the patient is allowed more activity in bed and is started on limited activity, progressing from short periods in a comfortable chair to short walks under supervision. Comparison of pulse rate, blood pressure, and respiratory rate before and after activity are good guides to advancement of activity. Between the second and third week, many patients are discharged from the hospital to limited activity at home. Daily physical conditioning in the form of gradually extended walks begin at about one month. In two or three months, most patients may return to work.

The patient with complications such as congestive heart failure, recurrent arrhythmias, or A-V block will progress more slowly. Recurrent arrhythmia or A-V block will require a longer period of monitoring in the CCU before progressing to convalescent care. The patient who has experienced congestive heart failure or shock has extensive myocardial loss. His progress will be dictated by his response to gradually increasing activity. Survivors of complications such as a ruptured ventricular septum, papillary muscle, or ventricular aneurysm will require surgical intervention. Coronary arteriograms and saphenous-vein bypass grafts may be indicated in some patients following their recovery from the acute myocardial infarction.

An organized activities and educational program carried on while the patient is hospitalized can be an effective initial rehabilitation program. Such a program is outlined on the following pages.

ST. PATRICK HOSPITAL
Missoula, Montana 59801

PHYSICIANS ORDERS - MI REHAB

DATE	DIAGNOSIS _____ ALLERGIES WEIGHT	NURSE'S INITIAL AND TIME

1. PHYSICAL ACTIVITIES: (Each level to be ordered, separately, signed and dated by physician.)

PHYSICAL THERAPY EXERCISE

WARD ACTIVITIES

Level 1. Supine 1 -Passive R.O.M. all limbs.
Supine 2- advance to active exercise-all limbs
except shoulders 5X.

Level 1. Feed self in bed, If B.P.
stable, raise head of bed. Commode,
Dangle with legs elevated.

_____ M.D.

Level 2-Active assistive upper and lower
extremity exercise-supine, Exercised #1-3
(Cardiac Rehab Home Exercise Program) to maximum of 25 counts.

Level 2. Passive shoulder exercises
Commode. Chair 2X, 10-20 minutes.
Partial a.m. self-care, wash hands, face,
brush teeth.

_____ M.D.

Level 3-Active exercise No. 1-3 as above

Level 3. Bath in bed(self) nurse to
do back and feet. Walk to bathroom
with assistance. Chair 3X daily,
20-30 minutes.

_____ M.D.

Level 4-Begin to add exercises starting with
No. 4&5, sitting and Supine X25 counts.

Level 4-Chair 3 or 4X per day. To
bathroom with assistance. Active
shoulder and hip.

_____ M.D.

Level 5-Continue to add exercises. Standing
X25 counts. Progress to maximum of 10 exercises X25 counts.

Level 5-Tub bath. Shave, comb hair,
brush teeth - standing

_____ M.D.

Level 6-To Physical Therapy Dept. Continue to
progress with exercises X25 counts. Begin am-
bulation.-50', Increase distance as indicated.

Level 6-Shower with assistance. Walk in
hall 2 or 3X.

_____ M.D.

Level 7-Continue with exercises as above. Continue to increase distance walking. If feasible
walk to PT Dept. with supervision. Try on stairs.

Level 7-Walk up and down 1/2 flight
stairs under doctor's supervision.
Home. First doctor's appointment.

_____ M.D.

OT consult for sexuality and energy saving techniques _____ M.D.

Upon transfer to 4E the MI Rehab Educational Program will be automatically instituted
as per protocol unless otherwise ordered by the physician. 4E Ward Secretary notify:

Pharmacy _____ Date notified
Social Services _____ Date notified
Physical Therapy _____ Date notified
Dietary _____ Date notified

NOTE: DISPENSING BY NON-PROPRIETARY NAME IS AUTHORIZED UNLESS OTHERWISE INDICATED

PHYSICIANS ORDERS - MI REHAB

Courtesy of St. Patrick Hospital—Missoula, Montana.

M.I. REHAB PHYSICIANS ORDERS

THE FOLLOWING IS TO BE INITIATED BY THE PATIENT'S R.N. TEACHING COORDINATOR AS **APPROPRIATE TO THE PATIENT.** (M.D. DELETE, INITIAL AND DATE ITEMS R.N. COORDIATOR IS **NOT** TO INITIATE)

1.   TEACHING

   a. Anatomy

   b. Stress

   c. Risk factors

   d. Angina

   e. Medications:

      1. Digoxin

      2. Inderal

      3. Diuretics

      4. Anticoagulants

      5. Antihypertensives

      6. Nitrates

      7. Others: _____

2. OCCUPATIONAL THERAPY REFERRAL FOR

   a. Energy saving activities

   b. Sexuality

3. SOCIAL SERVICES

   a. Financial counseling

   b. Family counseling

   c. Vocational counseling

4. DIETARY INSTRUCTION APPROPRIATE TO DIET ORDERS

Courtesy of St. Patrick Hospital—Missoula, Montana.

1. Anxiety occurs in patients with myocardial infarction because of:

    A. _____   *threats.*

    B. _____   *fear.*

---

2. Anxiety may alter cardiac function by causing:

    A. ____ Tachycardia.   *A*

    B. ____ Hypertension.   *B*

    C. ____ Increased myocardial work.   *C*

    D. ____ Increased myocardial oxygen consumption.   *D*

---

3. Hostility, anger, or denial of illness may be early signs of _____.   *depression.*

---

4. A patient in a CCU becomes agitated and restless, resentful because he has to be fed, and angry at the night nurse because she takes his blood pressure. His major problem may be:

    A. ____ He thinks he is strong enough to feed himself.

    B. ____ He is cranky by nature.

    C. ____ He doesn't like the looks of the night nurse.

    D. ____ He fears he may die.   *D*

5. List ways the nurse may relieve a patient's anxiety and hostility:

    A. _____

    B. _____

    C. _____

    D. _____

    Optimism

    Reassurance

    Talking with the patient about fears

    Explanations to the patient

---

6. The patient who has just been admitted to the CCU does not want his wife called because he is afraid she will be worried. He is projecting his own _____ .

    fears

---

7. The patient is having electrodes attached and asks what they are for. He should be told:

    A. ____ "They will tell the nurse when your heart stops."

    B. ____ "They record the electro-cardiogram so that problems can be avoided."

    C. ____ "Quit worrying. The doctor knows best."

    B

---

8. The wife of a patient being monitored in the CCU exhibits considerable anxiety when she sees the strange equipment. Her husband has had no complications.

    She should be:

    A. ____ Warned that a high percentage of patients in the CCU have major fatal arrhythmias.

    B. ____ Reassured that the equipment is used to recognize major problems before they become serious.

    C. ____ Told that she can only stay for five minutes as her anxiety will disturb her husband.

    B

SUGGESTED READING—CHAPTER 14

1. Hackett, T. P., Cassem, N. H. and Wishner, H. A.: The coronary care unit: an appraisal of its psychologic hazards. *N. Eng. J. Med., 279,* 1365, 1968.

2. Hackett, T. P., Cassem, N. H. and Wishner, H. A.: Detection and treatment of anxiety in the coronary care unit. *Amer. Heart J., 78,* 727, 1969.

3. Druss, R. G. and Kornfeld, D. S.: The survivors of cardiac arrest. *J. Amer. Med. Assn., 201,* 291, 1967.

4. Parker, D. L. and Hodge, J. R.: Delirium in a coronary care unit. *J. Amer. Med. Assn., 201,* 702, 1967.

5. Swan, H. J. C., Blackburn, H. W., DeSanctis, R., Frommer, P. L., Hurst, J. W., Paul, O., Rapaport, E., Wallace, A. and Weinberg, S: Duration of hospitalization in "uncomplicated completed acute myocardial infarction." *Amer. J. Cardiol., 37,* 413, 1976.

6. Rose, G.: Early mobilization and discharge after myocardial infarction. *Mod. Concepts Cardiovasc. Dis., 41,* 59, 1972.

15

Special nursing procedures

The following nursing duties, though not necessarily peculiar to the coronary care unit, are important since they are done so commonly.

A. NURSING CARE OF PATIENT WITH MYOCARDIAL INFARCTION
B. A ROUTE FOR INTRAVENOUS MEDICATION
C. SKIN CARE TO PREVENT PHLEBITIS FROM INTRAVENOUS CATHETER
D. LEG WRAPPING
E. NURSING PROCEDURE FOR CENTRAL VENOUS AND PULMONARY ARTERY PRESSURE MONITORING
F. NURSING PROCEDURE FOR INSERTION OF A PACING CATHETER
G. NURSING PROCEDURE FOR A TRANSVENTRICULAR PACING ELECTRODE
H. NURSING PROCEDURE FOR ARTERIAL BLOOD SAMPLING

A. OUTLINE FOR NURSING CARE OF THE PATIENT WITH MYOCARDIAL INFARCTION

The details of nursing care of the patient with a myocardial infarction depend upon the severity of the infarction, the presence or absence of arrhythmias, shock, congestive failure, and complicating illnesses.

Immediate nursing care of the patient not in acute distress.

1. Start I.V. drip.
2. Attach monitor and obtain rhythm strip.
3. Relieve pain.
4. Examination:
   a. Skin: Pallor, cyanosis, moisture, temperature, edema.
   b. Neck veins.
   c. Cough and dyspnea.
   d. Mental status.
5. Obtain vital signs:
   a. Blood pressure. Note position of patient and which arm is used.
   b. Apical rate and rhythm. If irregular, check monitor, and compare with radial pulse rate.
   c. Respiratory rate and character.
6. Check history of medications and other diseases.
7. Observe other orders.
8. Undress patient.
9. Order lab work.
10. Explain the coronary care unit and need for rest.
11. Explain each new procedure before it is done.
12. Arrange a private conference with the family to explain the coronary care unit, treatment program, and visiting policy.

Immediate nursing care of the patient in acute distress (arrhythmias, pulmonary edema, shock).

1. Start I.V. drip.
2. Attach monitor and obtain rhythm strip.
3. Position patient for comfort.
4. Relieve pain.
5. Start oxygen.

6. Notify physician of above.
7. Check emergency equipment.
    a. Defibrillator.
    b. Cardiopulmonary resuscitation equipment.
    c. Rotating tourniquets.
8. Other measures as indicated for the patient *not in acute distress.*

B. A ROUTE FOR INTRAVENOUS MEDICATION

Purpose: The experienced CCU nurse does not feel at ease with a newly-admitted patient until she has a route available for emergency medication. During the early minutes after admission, the nurse may need to give morphine, lidocaine, atropine, Isuprel®, or sodium bicarbonate.

> The intravenous route is chosen because it allows rapid response and precise adjustment of the dose of the medication. In addition, it bypasses some disadvantages of oral medication such as vomiting.

The intravenous technique which is used must be *secure.* It must be available when needed most, as after precordial shock, during cardiopulmonary resuscitation, or usual movements in bed. It must be usable for several days. It should not unduly restrict the patient's movement in bed.

The right arm and the antecubital veins should be avoided; they should be preserved for possible insertion of a flow-directed balloon catheter.

Equipment

Modified scalp vein infusion set (Abbott No. 4590): A short needle with a short bevel and no hub may be taped securely on the forearm or hand. It may be used for a slow I.V. drip, or, with appropriate tubing and a plug, may be filled with heparin solution between injections of medication.

Plastic intravenous catheter ("Intracath," "Infusor"): The plastic intravenous catheter has proven most popular since it is easy to introduce and commonly can remain in place for three or more days, after which a nonbacterial phlebitis usually requires its removal.

TECHNIQUE FOR INSERTING THE "INFUSOR"

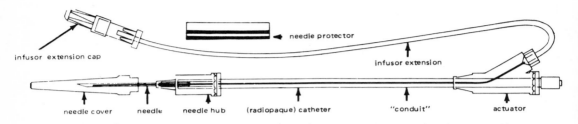

infusor extension cap

needle protector

infusor extension

needle cover needle needle hub (radiopaque) catheter "conduit" actuator

Description of Infusor

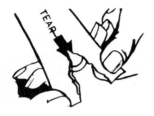

TEAR

1. Outer protective sack
   is opened.

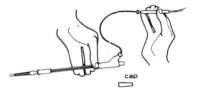

cap

2. Cap removed from end of
   extension tube and I.V.
   set is attached.

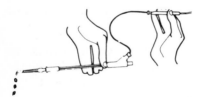

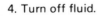

3. Flush catheter with solution.

4. Turn off fluid.

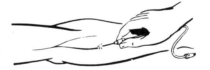

5. Make venipuncture in the usual
   way. Try to stay at least two
   inches distal to the elbow.

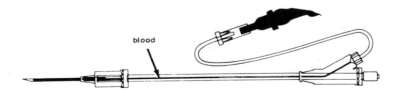

blood

6. Blood in the catheter may easily be seen through the
   translucent conduit.

C. SKIN CARE TO PREVENT PHLEBITIS AND INFECTION FROM A PLASTIC INTRAVENOUS CATHETER

Purpose: Meticulous skin care is worthwhile to minimize phlebitis and infection.

Technique

1. Use sterile gloves, mask, towels for drape, razor, basin, and water.
2. Shave site, using 15 cc. water plus 15 cc. pHisoHex.
3. Scrub 5 minutes with pHisoHex solution.
4. Scrub with aqueous Zephiran 1:750.
5. Introduce the needle and the catheter.
6. Apply firm pressure with sterile gauze pledget. When the needle is withdrawn over the catheter, blood seeps out, providing a fine locus for bacterial multiplication. Minimize this hematoma by firm pressure when the needle is withdrawn.
7. Anchor the catheter as usual, but do not get the nonsterile tape close to the point of entry.
8. Apply a small dab of Neosporin or Betadine ointment to the entry site and cover with sterile gauze.
9. Write date and time on the dressing.
10. Apply dressing in such a way that the puncture site can be attended daily.
11. Each day, remove the gauze pledget, wipe the site with dry gauze, and apply a small dab of antibiotic ointment and a new gauze pledget.
12. Notify the physician if phlebitis or local inflammation is apparent.
13. If pus appears, culture, and notify physician. If the catheter is removed, culture the catheter tip by cutting off the distal two inches and dropping it into a culture tube containing broth.

D. LEG WRAPPING

Purpose: Leg wrapping is done to prevent thrombi in the leg veins and thereby reduce the likelihood of pulmonary emboli.

On first thought, it might seem strange to wrap the legs to prevent venous clotting. However, the significant thrombus which might break loose and be carried to the lungs is a thrombus in the internal or *deep* leg veins adjacent to the bones.

A factor which will speed the flow of blood in the deep veins will reduce the chance of thrombus formation. Occlusion of the superficial veins with elastic bandages or stockings will direct more blood through the deep veins, increasing the flow rate.

Many doctors hesitate to order leg wrapping since a poorly performed wrapping or poorly-fitting stockings only produce local constriction and discomfort. For effectiveness, compression should decrease gradually from foot to knee. For safety, there must be no zone of tight constriction; tight constriction is nothing more than a garter which impedes deep venous flow and tends to cause rather than prevent thrombosis.

Technique

1. Use two 3-inch elastic bandages for each leg.
2. Begin at the base of the toes, overlapping $^4/_5$, keeping the bandage fairly snug.
3. On ascending the leg, wrap looser and use less overlap, resulting in about ½ overlap on the calf.
4. Stop just below the knee.
5. Place a strip of adhesive tape down each side of the leg wrapping to help keep it in place.
6. Inspect wrappings for smoothness at least every 8 hours.
7. Rewrap when any disorder appears, or every 12 hours.

E. NURSING PROCEDURE FOR CENTRAL VENOUS AND PULMONARY ARTERY PRESSURE MONITORING

(An asterisk indicates those steps usually performed by the physician.)

1. Prepare the skin over the vein to be used.
*2. Introduce a polyethylene catheter into the vein (via a cutdown or through a needle).
*3. Advance the catheter into the vena cava or right atrium.
4. Connect the catheter to a three-way stopcock, which in turn is connected to a manometer and to a bottle of parenteral fluid, most commonly 5% glucose in water.
5. Fill the manometer with fluid from the I.V. bottle.
6. Determine the location of the right atrium. Ordinarily, the right atrium is assumed to be 5 cm. dorsal to the level at which the second costal cartilage joins the sternum. Mark this point with a small piece of tape on the side of the chest. Using a carpenter's spirit level, adjust the position of the manometer so that the 0 point is equal to the central venous pressure.

7. After a reading has been obtained, turn the stopcock so that the fluid in the I.V. bottle is connected with the catheter to keep the system open and free of clots.

8. The patient should be supine and the bed should be flat when measurements of CVP are made.

Insertion of a flow-directed balloon catheter for recording pulmonary diastolic or "wedge" pressure is similar to insertion of a CVP catheter. The catheter is introduced via a cutdown and advanced to the right atrium, where the balloon is inflated. Connection is made to a manometer or pressure recorder, then advanced to the pulmonary artery. *The balloon should not remain inflated between wedge pressure recordings since it occludes the artery.* The catheter is maintained open by a drip of heparinized solution or a heparin lock.

F. NURSING PROCEDURE FOR INSERTION OF A PACING CATHETER

(Using Endocardial ECG as a Guide to Location of the Catheter Tip)

Purpose

1. Diagnosis of arrhythmias by demonstrating large P waves in the ECG recorded from within the right atrium.
2. Heart pacing.

Technique (An asterisk indicates those steps usually performed by the physician.)

1. Administer sedative or other pre-op medication if ordered.
2. Collect all necessary equipment at the bedside.
3. Disconnect electrical equipment, other than ECG (or insure a common ground for multiple items of electrical apparatus).
4. Apply ECG electrodes to each of the four extremities, using abrasive ECG electrode paste (not cream).
5. Shave and prepare the skin of the site to be used (the subclavian vein in the infraclavicular area; the jugular vein at the side of the neck; the basilic vein at the antecubital fossa; the femoral vein below the inguinal ligament).
*6. Don rubber gloves for insulation.
*7. Drape the area of venipuncture and place a large drape over the trunk, to receive the long and floppy pacing catheter.

*8.   Infiltrate over the vein with lidocaine.

*9.   Insert a plastic needle, remove the metal stylet, and advance to the vein. (Surgical exposure of the vein may be necessary.)

*10.   Insert the pacing catheter through the plastic needle.

11.   Attach the distal end of the pacing catheter to the chest lead wire (V lead) of ECG cable, using alligator clips on the connecting cable.

12.   Put the ECG lead selector switch on "V." Watch ECG pattern as catheter is advanced (into the atrium for arrhythmia diagnosis, or into the right ventricle for pacing).

13.   Judge the location of the tip from the appearance of P and QRS as described below.

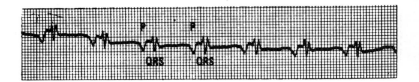

Innominate vein: The ECG resembles a unipolar extremity lead. The P wave is inverted. It becomes a greater amplitude as the catheter tip approaches the atrium.

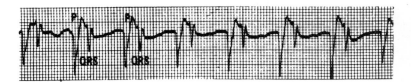

High right atrium: When the tip of the catheter enters the right atrium, the P wave becomes quite large, often larger than QRS. The exact form of the P wave varies with catheter position within the atrium. Recording from high in the atrium (above the sinus node), the P is negative.

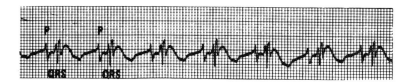

Low right atrium: The P wave is large and either positive or diphasic (positive-negative).

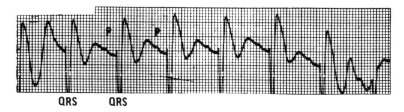

Right ventricle: As the catheter enters the right ventricle, the P wave becomes small and remains positive, similar to a record from a V lead recorded from the chest wall. The QRS becomes very large. In the right ventricle the QRS fundamentally is negative, but usually there is a small initial R wave.

If advanced into the **pulmonary artery,** the P and QRS again resemble aVR or aVL or perhaps lead V1 or V2, both in size and configuration.

If the catheter enters the *coronary sinus* instead of the right ventricle, a large "atrial" type of P wave will be recorded. Though the QRS may change somewhat, it will not be the large negative complex expected in a right ventricular recording.

14. Watch the oscilloscope for ectopic beats. When the catheter tip is in the ventricle, VPC's or runs of ventricular tachycardia are common. Be prepared to treat with I.V. lidocaine or precordial shock. (Pronounced ST elevation is common when the tip is pressing against the ventricular wall.)

*15. If a unipolar catheter is used, an indifferent electrode is needed. Infiltrate the skin of precordium or near the venipuncture site with lidocaine. Place an indifferent electrode suture here. Break off the straight needle at the other end of the indifferent electrode so that it is ½ inch long. Attach the indifferent electrode to the positive pole of the pulse generator and the distal end of the pacemaker catheter to the negative pole of the pulse generator.

16. Set the pulse generator current at about 1.5 ma, rate usually about 70.
17. Advise the patient that he may feel some electrical sensations near the indifferent electrode suture.
18. Turn on the pulse generator.
19. Gradually advance the amplitude of the current to determine the threshold.
*20. If satisfactory capture is obtained, remove the plastic needle from the arm, leaving the pacing catheter in place.
*21. Fix the catheter to the skin with silk suture.
22. Apply gauze dressing to the venipuncture site.
23. Strap the pulse generator to the body and arrange the indifferent electrode and the pacing catheter so that they cannot be dislodged accidentally.

Equipment Needed

Insertion of the Pacing Catheter Using Endocardial ECG as a Guide to Location of the Catheter Tip

Occasionally this procedure must be done with minimum personnel and minimum loss of time. Therefore, it is helpful to have a large sterile package ("pacing kit") containing the sterile goods which can be autoclaved. While the nurse is preparing the arm, the doctor puts on mask and gown, scrubs, and arranges the sterile goods on the table.

1. Masks and caps for all personnel.
2. Scrub brush.
3. Doctor's gowns.
4. Skin prep equipment.
5. Lidocaine, 10 ml. of 1% solution (100 mg.) for possible I.V. use.
6. Venous cannulation equipment including at least the following:
    a. Four towels
    b. Large drape
    c. Small drape with hole
    d. Four towel clips
    e. Suture scissors, rat-tooth forceps, needle holder
    f. Scalpel blade, No. 11
7. Connecting cable, V lead to catheter: Two feet of flexible, insulated wire with a small battery clip at one end and a large battery clip at the other end.

8. Longdwell needle, which will accept a bipolar catheter.

9. Emergency percutaneous transventricular pacing needle with wire.

10. Pacing catheter: Elecath No. 560 Semifloating Unipolar Pacemaker Catheter, 4F, 100 cm. (Electro-Catheter Corporation, 249 Wescott Drive, Rahway, N.J., 07065).

11. Jelco I.V. Catheter Placement Needle, 14 gauge, 2½ inch (Electro-Catheter Corporation).

12. NBIH—Bipolar Pacemaking Catheter: U.S.C.I., No. 5651, 5F, 100 cm. (United States Catheter and Instrument Company, P.O. Box 787, Glens Falls, New York, 12801).

13. Indifferent electrode: Flexon stainless steel, multistrand 24-inch suture with straight cutting needle on one end and ½ circle taper needle on opposite end (Davis and Geck, No. 12597-63).

14. ECG limb electrodes.

15. Abrasive paste (Redux Electrode Paste, Hewlett-Packard Company, Order No. 651-1008).

16. Five-wire ECG cable.

17. Monitoring device, either bedside oscilloscope or ECG instrument, properly grounded.

18. Defibrillator (at the bedside, turned on but not charged), tongue blade, and abrasive electrode paste.

19. Equipment for cardiopulmonary resuscitation.

20. Pulse generator.

G. NURSING PROCEDURE FOR A TRANSVENTRICULAR PACING ELECTRODE

Purpose: To provide a method of delivering a pacemaking stimulus to the ventricle with minimum delay.

Technique (An asterisk indicates those steps usually performed by the physician.)

1. Assemble all necessary equipment at the bedside.

2. Prepare the skin widely from the xiphoid process to the left axilla.

3. Drape.

*4. Infiltrate the skin with lidocaine and nick with a scalpel blade.

*5. *Right Ventricular Approach*
    a. Introduce the needle and its contained fishhook wire just to the left of the xiphoid, in about the sixth intercostal space.
    b. Aim medial, cephalad, and dorsal at an angle of 30 degrees to the skin (aim at the second right costochondral junction).

*6. *Left Ventricular Approach*
    a. Insert the needle and its contained fishhook wire at the point of maximum impulse (cardiac apex).
    b. Aim toward the right shoulder.

*7. Advance until the ventricular impulse is felt, then one or two cm. further until ventricular blood is obtained.

*8. Withdraw the needle over wire. The fishhook protrusion will impinge on the endocardium.

9. Connect the myocardial wire to the negative pole of the pulse generator.

*10. Suture the indifferent electrode wire to the skin over the precordium and connect to the positive pole of the pulse generator.

11. Secure the myocardial wire to the skin, with tape or suture.

12. Be prepared to treat VPC's or ventricular tachycardia with I.V. lidocaine or with precordial shock.

Equipment Needed for a Pacing Electrode

1. No. 18 thin wall needle, 6 inches long, containing an 18-inch length of 32 gauge (size zero) stainless steel suture protruding ¼ inch beyond the tip of the needle, bent over as a fishhook.

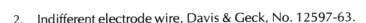

2. Indifferent electrode wire, Davis & Geck, No. 12597-63.
3. Defibrillator.
4. Skin prep material.
5. Rubber gloves and masks for all personnel.
6. Scalpel blade, No. 11.
7. Towels and drapes.
8. Lidocaine.

H. NURSING PROCEDURE FOR ARTERIAL BLOOD SAMPLING

Purpose: To obtain arterial blood for one or more of the following tests: oxygen, carbon dioxide, or pH.

Normal values

> pH: 7.38–7.42
> Oxygen saturation: 97% or more
> PaCO$_2$: 30–40 mm. Hg.

Indications

A. To evaluate lung function in removal of carbon dioxide from, and addition of oxygen to, blood.
1. Blood in the veins already has passed through the capillaries, taking up carbon dioxide and giving up oxygen to the body tissues. Therefore, the oxygen, carbon dioxide, and acid (pH) content of *venous* blood is determined by body cell activity as well as by lung function.
2. Arterial sampling permits study of blood before it has been altered by circulation through the capillaries. (See sketch)
B. To determine if unoxygenated blood is leaking into the arterial circuit from the right side of the heart through a congenital defect.

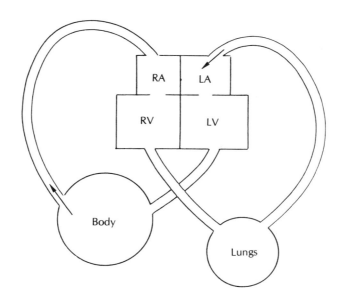

Equipment Needed

1. Arterial blood tray:
   a. Cournand needle & 219 × 1'' needle
   b. Plastic syringes
   c. Drapes
   d. Needles & syringes for local anesthesia
2. Gloves, three pair.
3. Masks for all personnel.
4. Plastic sheet (to protect linen).
5. Folded bath blanket (to provide hyperextension of elbow or wrist).
6. Lidocaine, 1%, 30 cc. vial.
7. Oxygen.
8. Oxygen mask with rebreathing bag.
9. One pint of ice cubes in a one-quart can or pitcher.
10. Kling, 3 inch, nonsterile.
11. Skin prep tray.
12. Mercury in a syringe.

Procedure: After arterial puncture, blood is collected in heparinized syringes. Mercury may be added to permit the lab to mix the blood prior to analysis. The syringes immediately are placed in ice water to stop blood cell metabolism, which otherwise would alter the blood. Oxygen then may be administered by mask to test the lung's ability to increase oxygen transfer to the blood. After removal of the needle, the puncture site is compressed firmly by hand for five minutes to prevent leakage of blood from the artery.

Those steps marked by an asterisk may be done by the physician.

1. Explain purpose and procedure to the patient.
2. Remove the gown from the arm to be used.
3. Place a folded bath blanket beneath the elbow. (Hyperextension makes the brachial artery more superficial. The radial artery also may be used as a sampling site.)
4. Place a plastic sheet between the arm and the bath blanket.
5. Place a nonsterile towel between the arm and the plastic sheet.
6. Put on a mask.
7. Scrub the site with a mixture of water and pHisoHex or equivalent.
8. Scrub with Tr. Merthiolate or equivalent.
*9. Drape with sterile towels.
*10. Infiltrate lidocaine over the artery.

*11.   Introduce a needle into the artery.

12.   Call the laboratory to receive blood samples.

*13.   Expel air bubble from the sample.

*14.   Add mercury to the sample.

15.   Cap the syringe.

*16.   Remove the needle.

17.   Compress the brachial puncture site for five minutes firmly enough to obliterate the radial pulse.

18.   Apply Kling and a wad of 2×2 gauze over the puncture site; wrap firmly, but do not obliterate the radial pulse.

19.   Remove the pressure dressing in ten minutes. The arm may lie in a horizontal position.

20.   Observe for bleeding, hematoma, and presence of radial pulse. If radial pulse is absent, notify physician stat; continue observation for at least ten minutes. Avoid this arm for blood pressure monitoring for at least 4 hours.

Record Keeping

Complete laboratory requisitions as ordered.
Note which arm was used.
Note presence or absence of hematoma, bleeding, and radial pulse.

SUGGESTED READING—CHAPTER 15

1. Hamilton, A. J.: *Selected Subjects for Critical Care Nurses.* Mountain Press Publishing Company, Missoula, Mt., 1975.

2. Alpert, J. S. and Francis, G. S.: *Manual of Coronary Care.* Little, Brown and Company, Boston, 1977.

3. Meltzer, L. E. and Dunning, A. J.: *Textbook of Coronary Care.* The Charles Press, Philadelphia, 1972.

Appendix

For your convenience, the following charts and tables have been repeated in the appendix. They are designed to be removed from the book and posted in a convenient place in the CCU.

Flow Diagram: Management of Myocardial Infarction
A Summary of Arrhythmias
Cardiovascular Drugs

MANAGEMENT OF MYOCARDIAL INFARCTION

| Prompt professional response to reported symptoms. Trained ambulance personnel. Prompt transfer to hospital. Prompt admission to ICCF. | → | If symptoms suspicious enough to warrant hospitalization, immediate ICC needed. | Monitor. Start I.V. (to provide route for urgent medication). Defibrillator at bedside, ready to use. Write orders for routine and emergency measures. |

CONGESTIVE HEART FAILURE?

↓

Oxygen.
Diuretics.
Digoxin (I.V., fractional doses).
Sodium restriction.
Monitor pulmonary
   artery pressure or wedge
   pressure.
Edecrin® or Lasix® I.V.
Vasodilators.

PULMONARY EDEMA?

↓

Morphine I.V.
Oxygen.
Rotating tourniquets.
Phlebotomy?
Dangle.
Digoxin I.V.
Edecrin® or Lasix® I.V.
Follow PCWP carefully.

SHOCK?

↓

Monitor pulmonary
   artery pressure or wedge
   pressure.
If PCWP low or normal, consider
   fluid replacement with
   repeated challenge doses.
Monitor hourly urine volume.
Determine position which
   provides maximum comfort
   and maximum BP.
Recall unreliability of BP
   measurements.
Oxygen.
Consider dopamine.
Consider digoxin (especially if
   PCWP high).
Consider Levophed® or Aramine®.
Consider Vasodilators.

DIGITALIS TOXICITY?

↓

Check serum potassium and
   history of potassium
   intake and output.
Avoid precordial shock.
Consider lidocaine, quinidine
   or Pronestyl.®
Dilantin or Inderal® I.V., if
   ventricular arrhythmias.
Pace if A-V block results
   in serious fall in C.O.

FIRST DEGREE A-V HEART BLOCK?

↓

Try atropine, I.V.
Avoid morphine, if possible.
Hold digitalis.
Prepare pacing equipment.

SECOND DEGREE A-V HEART BLOCK?

↓

Atropine, I.V.
Consider transvenous pacing
   catheter.
Avoid quinidine, Pronestyl®,
   lidocaine, unless paced.

THIRD DEGREE A-V HEART BLOCK?

↓

Avoid quindine, Pronestyl®,
   lidocaine, unless paced.
Isuprel.®
Pacing catheter and demand
   pulse generator.
Don't hesitate to pace via
   percutaneous ventricular
   puncture if situation is urgent
   and transvenous catheterization
   not promptly successful.

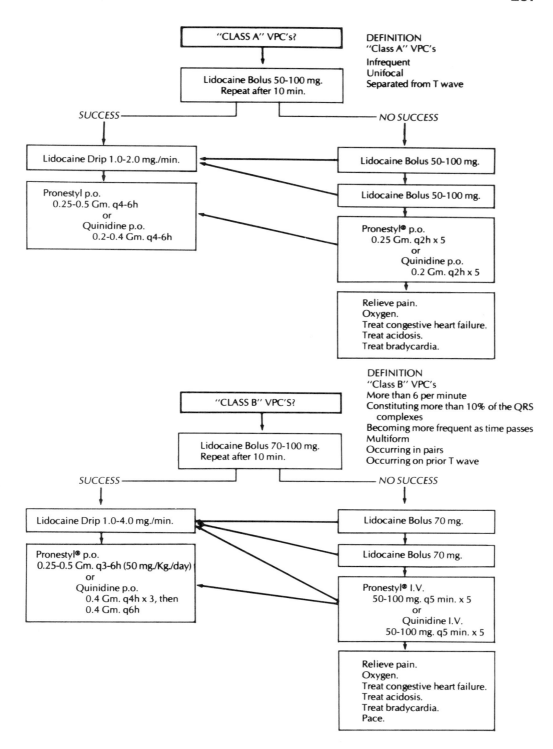

"CLASS A" VPC's?

Lidocaine Bolus 50-100 mg.
Repeat after 10 min.

DEFINITION
"Class A" VPC's
Infrequent
Unifocal
Separated from T wave

SUCCESS ——— *NO SUCCESS*

Lidocaine Drip 1.0-2.0 mg./min.

Lidocaine Bolus 50-100 mg.

Pronestyl p.o.
0.25-0.5 Gm. q4-6h
or
Quinidine p.o.
0.2-0.4 Gm. q4-6h

Lidocaine Bolus 50-100 mg.

Pronestyl® p.o.
0.25 Gm. q2h x 5
or
Quinidine p.o.
0.2 Gm. q2h x 5

Relieve pain.
Oxygen.
Treat congestive heart failure.
Treat acidosis.
Treat bradycardia.

DEFINITION
"Class B" VPC's
More than 6 per minute
Constituting more than 10% of the QRS
    complexes
Becoming more frequent as time passes
Multiform
Occurring in pairs
Occurring on prior T wave

"CLASS B" VPC'S?

Lidocaine Bolus 70-100 mg.
Repeat after 10 min.

SUCCESS ——— *NO SUCCESS*

Lidocaine Drip 1.0-4.0 mg./min.

Lidocaine Bolus 70 mg.

Pronestyl® p.o.
0.25-0.5 Gm. q3-6h (50 mg./Kg./day)
or
Quinidine p.o.
0.4 Gm. q4h x 3, then
0.4 Gm. q6h

Lidocaine Bolus 70 mg.

Pronestyl® I.V.
50-100 mg. q5 min. x 5
or
Quinidine I.V.
50-100 mg. q5 min. x 5

Relieve pain.
Oxygen.
Treat congestive heart failure.
Treat acidosis.
Treat bradycardia.
Pace.

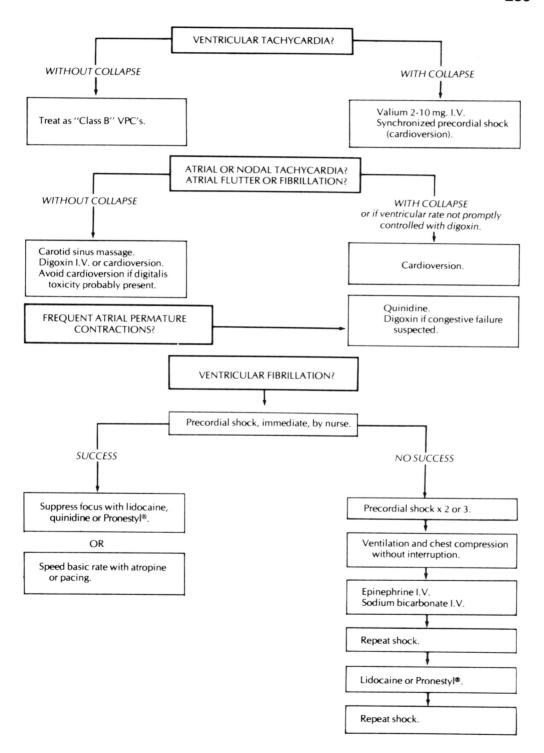

VENTRICULAR TACHYCARDIA?

WITHOUT COLLAPSE

Treat as "Class B" VPC's.

WITH COLLAPSE

Valium 2-10 mg. I.V.
Synchronized precordial shock
(cardioversion).

ATRIAL OR NODAL TACHYCARDIA?
ATRIAL FLUTTER OR FIBRILLATION?

WITHOUT COLLAPSE

Carotid sinus massage.
Digoxin I.V. or cardioversion.
Avoid cardioversion if digitalis
toxicity probably present.

FREQUENT ATRIAL PERMATURE
CONTRACTIONS?

WITH COLLAPSE
or if ventricular rate not promptly
controlled with digoxin.

Cardioversion.

Quinidine.
Digoxin if congestive failure
suspected.

VENTRICULAR FIBRILLATION?

Precordial shock, immediate, by nurse.

SUCCESS

Suppress focus with lidocaine,
quinidine or Pronestyl®.

OR

Speed basic rate with atropine
or pacing.

NO SUCCESS

Precordial shock x 2 or 3.

Ventilation and chest compression
without interruption.

Epinephrine I.V.
Sodium bicarbonate I.V.

Repeat shock.

Lidocaine or Pronestyl®.

Repeat shock.

A SUMMARY OF ARRHYTHMIAS

Rhythm	Significance	ECG	Treatment
SINUS BRADYCARDIA	Low cardiac output if stroke volume limited.	Rate less than 60. PR constant and normal.	Atropine, pacing.
SINUS TACHYCARDIA	Low cardiac output when filling time inadequate.	Rate more than 100. PR constant and normal.	Treat basic problem.
SINUS ARRHYTHMIA	Usually none.	PR constant and normal. Variable R-R interval.	None.
ATRIAL PREMATURE CONTRACTIONS	Often indicate congestive failure. May lead to other atrial arrhythmias.	Premature P with different configuration.	None, or consider quinidine or digitalis.
ATRIAL TACHYCARDIA	Cardiac output may fall. Suggests digitalis toxicity.	P often hidden. Ventricular rhythm regular. Rate about 200.	Carotid pressure, digitalis, cardioversion, Tensilon.
ATRIAL FLUTTER	Often indicates congestive failure. Cardiac output may fall.	Flutter waves, 300 per minute. Usually 2:1, 3:1, 4:1 or variable A-V conduction.	Cardioversion, digitalis.
ATRIAL FIBRILLATION	Often indicates congestive failure. Cardiac output may fall.	Fibrillation waves, 350-500/min., with variable contour.	Digitalis, cardioversion.

Rhythm	Significance	ECG	Treatment
JUNCTIONAL PREMATURE CONTRACTIONS	Same as APC's.	Ventricular rhythm irregular. Inverted P precedes, is buried in, or follows QRS.	Same as APC's.
JUNCTIONAL TACHYCARDIA	Sames as atrial tachycardia. Suggests digitalis toxicity	Inverted P precedes, is buried in, or follows, QRS.	Sames as atrial tachycardia.
VENTRICULAR PREMATURE CONTRACTIONS	May lead to ventricular tachycardia or fibrillation.	QRS premature, broad, "different" and not preceded by premature P.	Lidocaine, quinidine, Pronestyl®
VENTRICULAR TACHYCARDIA	Often progresses to vascular collapse or ventricular fibrillation.	QRS broad. Ventricular rhythm nearly regular. P unrelated to QRS. Average rate 180.	Lidocaine, quinidine, Pronestyl®, cardioversion.
VENTRICULAR FIBRILLATION	No cardiac output. Fatal if untreated.	No well-defined QRS. Irregular undulations.	Precordial shock.
FIRST DEGREE A-V BLOCK	May progress to higher degree block. May indicate excess quinidine, Pronestyl®, or digitalis.	PR 0.21 sec. or more. Each P conducted.	Observe for higher degree block.
SECOND DEGREE A-V BLOCK	May progress to complete block.	Some P waves not conducted.	Insert pacemaker catheter. Atropine.
THIRD DEGREE A-V BLOCK	Low cardiac output. May produce shock, congestive failure, syncope, ventricular arrhythmias.	P unrelated to QRS. Ventricular rate 20-45. QRS narrow or broad.	Pacemaker. Isuprel® may speed ventricular rate, but used only temporarily.

CARDIOVASCULAR DRUGS

Drug	Usual Dose	Uses	Toxicity
LANOXIN® DIGOXIN	Digitalizing dose: 2.0-3.0 mg. orally; 1.0-2.0 mg. I.V.	Congestive heart failure, control ventricular rate in atrial flutter or fibrillation.	VPC's, A-V conduction disturbances, nausea, vomiting, yellow vision, and other CNS symptoms.
DIGITOXIN	Digitalizing dose: 1.0-2.0 mg. orally.	Same as digoxin but slower action and more prolonged effect.	Same as digoxin; toxicity more prolonged.
XYLOCAINE® LIDOCAINE	70-100 mg. I.V. x 3; 1.0-4.0 mg/min. I.V. drip.	Ventricular arrhythmias.	Seizures, A-V block.
PRONESTYL® PROCAINAMIDE	0.5 Gm. q 6 h orally; 50-100 mg. I.V. q 5 min. x 5.	Atrial and ventricular arrhythmias.	Hypotension, diarrhea, intraventricular con- duction delay, ventricular arrhythmias, skin rash, systemic lupus erythematosis.
QUINIDINE	0.2-0.4 Gm. q 4 h orally; 100 mg. I.V. q 5 min. x 5.	Atrial and ventricular arrhythmias.	GI symptoms, tinnitus, fever, syncope, thrombo- cytopenia, hypotension, intraventricular con- duction delay, ventricular arrhythmias.
BRETYLOL® BRETYLIUM TOSYLATE	5 mg./kg. I.V. over 8 minute period or I.M. Increase to 10 mg./kg. at 15-30 min. intervals up to 30 mg./kg.	Ventricular tachycardia or ventricular fibrillation.	Hypotension with low dose, nausea, vomiting, bradycardia, angina.

Drug	Usual Dose	Uses	Toxicity
DILANTIN® DIPHENYLHYDANTOIN	250 mg., diluted in 5 cc. solution, I.V. slowly over 5 min.; 100 mg. q.i.d. orally.	Arrhythmias due to digitalis toxicity. Prophylactically prior to cardioversion.	Local thrombophlebitis. Respiratory arrest.
INDERAL® PROPRANOLOL	10–80 mg. q 6 h orally; 0.5–1.0 mg./min. I.V.	Atrial and ventricular arrhythmias, angina.	Heart failure, shock, asthma, A-V block.
ATROPINE	0.5–1.0 mg./min. I.V.	Sinus bradycardia, A-V block.	May slow ventricular rate in 2° A-V block, glaucoma, urinary retention, delirium, fever.
ISUPREL® ISOPROTERENOL	0.2–1.0 mg. in 500 cc. I.V. drip.	Bradycardia, third degree A-V block.	Tachycardia, ventricular arrhythmias, myocardial necrosis.
EPINEPHRINE	1.0 mg. (1 cc. of 1:1000) I.V.	Ventricular fibrillation when no response to precordial shock.	Tachycardia, ventricular arrhythmias.
SODIUM BICARBONATE, 7.5%	50 cc. initially, repeated every 5 min. of circulatory arrest.	Correction of accidosis due to circulatory arrest or shock.	Local thrombophlebitis, sodium excess.

Drug	Usual Dose	Uses	Toxicity
EDECRIN® ETHACRYNIC ACID	25–50 mg. I.V., 50–400 mg. orally in divided doses.	Acute pulmonary edema, congestive heart failure, hypertension.	Potassium depletion, alkalosis, excess diuresis, acute gout, thrombocytopenia.
LASIX® FUROSEMIDE	10–80 mg. I.V.; 40–320 mg. orally.	Same as ethacrynic acid.	Potassium depletion, alkalosis, excess diuresis.
INTROPIN® DOPAMINE HCl	2–5 mcg./kg./min. initially, increase q 10 min. to desired effect. Dosage over 30 mcg./kg./min. acts like norepinephrine.	Shock, chronic congestive heart failure.	Ectopic beats, nausea, vomiting, tachycardia, angina.
GLUCAGON	2.5–5.0 mg. I.V. infusion, 1–4 mcg./kg./min.	Shock, acute heart failure, especially where propranolol has been used.	Nausea, hypoglycemia, hypokalemia.
ARAMINE® METARAMINOL	50–200 mg./L; give 2–3 cc./min. I.V.	Shock.	Uses body's own catecholamines so may need increasing dose, ventricular arrhythmias, excessive vasopressor response persists 20–60 min.
LEVOPHED® NOREPINEPHRINE	1–4 ampules (4–16 mg. Levophed base) per liter, 20–30 drops per min.	Shock.	Cutaneous necrosis (treat with Regitine), reduction of blood volume, ventricular arrhythmias.
WYAMINE-® MEPHENTERMINE	1000 mg./L.; give 1-3 cc./min.	Shock.	CNS stimulation.

Drug	Usual Dose	Uses	Toxicity
NIPRIDE® SODIUM NITROPRUSSIDE	0.5–8 mcg./kg./min. Must be protected from light and not kept or used over 4 hours.	Hypertension, congestive heart failure.	Nausea, sweating, headache, angina, palpitation.
ALDOMET® METHYLDOPA	250–500 mg. q 6–8 hr. I.V. or PO.	Hypertension.	Somnolence, Parkinsonism.
APRESOLINE® HYDRALAZINE	25–100 mg. PO q 6 h.	Hypertension, congestive heart failure.	Postural hypotension, peripheral neuritis, blood dyscrasias, lupus erythematosis.
NITROGLYCERIN	Tablet—.3–.6 mg. sublingually 2–3 times. I.V.—8–80 mcg./min., average 30 mg./min. Paste—½–2 inches q 4–6 hr.	Angina, congestive heart failure.	Headache, tachycardia, hypotension.
ISORDIL® SORBITRATE® ISOSORBIDE DINITRATE	2.5–10 mg. q 4–6 hr.	Angina, congestive heart failure.	Headache, tachycardia, hypotension, nausea, vomiting.
MINIPRESS® PRAZOSIN HCl	1–5 mg. q 8 hr. PO.	Hypertension, congestive heart failure.	Hypotension, nausea, vomiting, fluid retention.
HEPARIN	5000–15,000 units I.V.; 10,000–20,000 units subcutaneously.	Decrease blood clotting tendency; prevent thrombi and emboli; control dose with clotting time.	Bleeding. Antidote: protamine sulfate or fresh blood.
COUMADIN® PANWARFIN® WARFARIN SODIUM	30–60 mg. initially, 2–10 mg. daily.	Same as heparin. Control dose with prothrombin time.	Bleeding. Antidote: Vitamin K (Mephyton®).

Index

Index of Illustrative Electrocardiograms

Date Due

BRODART, INC.   Cat. No. 23 233   Printed in U.S.A.